W9-CON-039

Assessing Clinical Reasoning: The Oral Examination and Alternative Methods

Assessing Clinical Reasoning: The Oral Examination and Alternative Methods

Elliott L. Mancall, M.D.
Philip G. Bashook, Ed.D.
Editors

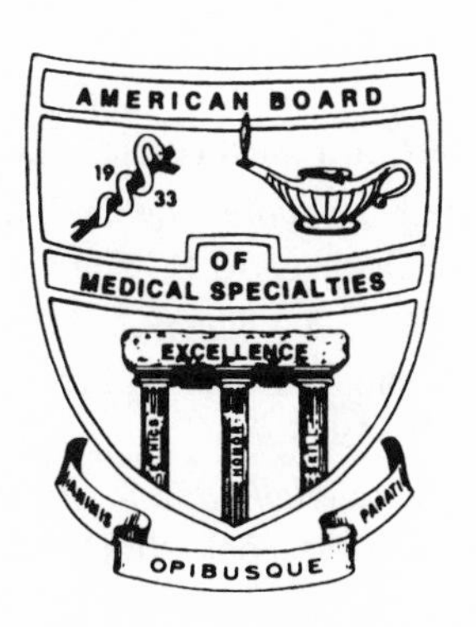

American Board of Medical Specialties
Evanston, Illinois
1995

Other Books Published by the American Board of Medical Specialties

Evaluation of Noncognitive Skills and Clinical Performance, Edited by John S. Lloyd, Ph.D., 1982.

Evaluating the Skills of Medical Specialists, Edited by John S. Lloyd, Ph.D., and Donald G. Langsley, M.D., 1983.

Oral Examinations in Medical Specialty Board Certification, Edited by John S. Lloyd, Ph.D., 1983.

Legal Aspects of Certification and Accreditation, Edited by Donald G. Langsley, M.D., 1983.

Computer Applications in the Evaluation of Physician Competence, Edited by John S. Lloyd, Ph.D., 1984.

Residency Director's Role in Specialty Certification, Edited by John S. Lloyd, Ph.D., 1985.

Trends in Specialization: Tomorrow's Medicine, Edited by Donald G. Langsley, M.D. and James H. Darragh, M.D., 1985.

Hospital Privileges and Specialty Medicine, Edited by Donald G. Langsley, M.D. and Mona M. Signer, 1986.

How to Evaluate Residents, Edited by John S. Lloyd, Ph.D. and Donald G. Langsley, M.D., 1986.

Recertification for Medical Specialists, Edited by John S. Lloyd, Ph.D. and Donald G. Langsley, M.D., 1987.

How to Select Residents, Edited by Donald G. Langsley, M.D., 1988.

Hospital Privileges and Specialty Medicine, 2nd Edition. Edited by Donald G. Langsley, M.D. and Beauregard Stubblefield, M.B.A., 1992.

Health Policy Issues Affecting Graduate Medical Education, Edited by Donald G. Langsley, M.D., J. Lee Dockery, M.D., and Peyton Weary, M.D., 1992.

The Ecology of Graduate Medical Education, Edited by Alexander J. Walt, M.B., Ch.B; Philip G. Bashook, Ed.D.; J. Lee Dockery, M.D.; Barbara S. Schneidman, M.D., M.P.H., 1993.

Recertification: New Evaluation Methods and Strategies, Edited by Elliott L. Mancall, M.D., and Philip G. Bashook, Ed.D., 1994.

ISBN: 0-934277-21-4

Library of Congress Catalog Card Number: 95-79294

Desktop publishing: Gail A. Strejc, American Board of Medical Specialties

Printed in the United States of America.

Contents

Preface

Sound reasoning and judgment are fundamental to effective functioning for all medical specialists and other professionals. The challenge in certifying professionals is ***how to assess reasoning?*** Since 1917 the Member Boards of the American Board of Medical Specialties (ABMS) have used oral examinations to evaluate the reasoning and judgment of board candidates. In fact, threads of controversy in medicine about the benefits, objectivity, and feasibility of large scale administration of oral examinations can be traced back through many years beginning with the round table meetings of the ABMS in 1941-1950, precursors of the current ABMS conferences. At ABMS conferences in 1975, and again in 1982, Member Boards reported on progress in developing and using standardized oral examinations.

These proceedings are from the ABMS conference held in Chicago on March 17, 1995, *Assessing Clinical Reasoning: If not the oral examination, what?* The conferences in 1975 and 1982 and this conference are a testament to the enduring interest in this examination method. Fifteen of the 24 ABMS Member Boards currently use standardized oral examinations for initial certification. Many other certification and licensure organizations, both within and outside of medicine, also use oral examinations. These proceedings provide an expanded look at the perceived contributions of oral examinations for assessing clinical reasoning, and address the issue as to whether newer evaluation methods might supplant this assessment method.

Recent advances in computer technology combined with studies on the reasoning processes of experts provide a solid foundation for a variety of new evaluation technologies. In light of these advances, half the conference was devoted to assessment of the current state-of-the-art in using *standardized* oral examinations to assess reasoning and judgment, while the remainder explored the potential role of newer technologies for assessing clinical reasoning and judgment. Among the newer technologies considered were:

- The "key features examination"
- Computerized patient simulations (CBX)
- Interstation patient notes used in objective structured clinical examinations (OSCEs)
- Assessment of commercial airline crews during simulated flights
- Computer-aided design (CAD) examinations in an architectural licensing examination.

The proceedings parallel the conference program as presented. **Maurice J. Martin, M.D.** (President of the American Board of Medical Specialties) welcomed participants by recalling the history of ABMS conferences and the long-standing emphasis on topics concerned with the quality of certification and training of physicians. **Elliott Mancall, M.D.** (conference moderator and COSEP Chairman) introduced the conference and presented a paper on the history of the oral examination in board certification in Part 1of this book. The keynote address by **Gordon G. Page, Ed.D.** (University of British Columbia, Canada) challenged the audience to think about both what to assess and how to assess clinical reasoning and judgment. (Part 2).

The remainder of the conference was structured into two sections: The oral examination, and alternatives to the oral examination. In the Proceedings Part 3 contains the papers from the session on *Potential value of the oral examination* by **Mary Ann Reinhart, Ph.D.** (American Board of Emergency Medicine) discussing the advantages of oral examinations, and by **Robert O. Guerin, Ph.D.** (American Board of Pediatrics) discussing the disadvantages, followed by a synopsis of the panel discussion. Part 4 includes papers by **Francis P. Hughes, Ph.D.**, (American Board of Anesthesiology), **Stephen C. Scheiber, M.D.**, (American Board of Psychiatry and Neurology), **Robert W. Cantrell, M.D. and Byron J. Bailey, M.D.**, (American Board of Otolaryngology), **Albert B. Gerbie, M.D. and William Droegemueller, M.D.**, (American Board of Obstetrics and Gynecology), **Philip G. Bashook, Ed.D.**, (American Board of Medical Specialties), and **Mary E. Lunz, Ph.D.**, (Board of Registry of the American College of Clinical Pathologists).

The second half of the conference began with a paper by **Isaac I. Bejar, Ph.D.** (Educational Testing Service, Princeton) describing a computer-based examination program for licensing architects. (Part 5). This was followed by a session on *alternatives to the standardized oral examination,* contained in Part 6, including papers by: **W. Dale Dauphinee, M.D.,** (Medical Council of Canada); **Stephen G. Clyman, M.D., Donald E. Melnick, M.D. and Brian E. Clauser, Ed.D.** (National Board of Medical Examiners); **Paula L. Stillman, M.D.**, (Medical College of Pennsylvania/Hahnemann University), **Youde Wang, Ph.D.**, (Eastern Virginia Medical School), **and Alfred E. Stillman, M.D.** (Crozer Chester Medical Center); and **Jacques Des Marchais, M.D.** (Universite' de Sherbrooke). Part 7 consists of the contribution by **William R. Taggart** (National Aeronautics and Space Administration/University of Texas/Federal Aviation

Administration's Crew Research Project), while Part 8 contains the concluding remarks by **Dr. Page**.

After reading these papers one may conclude that there are indeed newer technologies emerging to assess clinical reasoning, but that even after 80 years the oral examination, when standardized, continues to be the best currently available measurement tool for assessing the non-cognitive abilities and judgment of professionals.

Elliott L. Mancall, M.D.
Philip G. Bashook, Ed.D.
Editors

Acknowledgments

These conference proceedings were prepared to memorialize the papers and discussions presented at the March 17, 1995 conference on *Assessing Clinical Reasoning: If not the oral examination, what?* Conceived by the Committee on Study of Evaluation Procedures (COSEP) of the American Board of Medical Specialties (ABMS), the conference was planned by a subcommittee of COSEP: Francis P. Hughes, Ph.D., Elliott L. Mancall, M.D., Mary Ann Reinhart, Ph.D., and Philip G. Bashook, Ed.D. (ABMS staff). The conference success is due in large measure to the thoughtful and dedicated work of the planning committee members, the excellent presentations by the 16 conference faculty, and the insightful comments and discussions from the 140 conference registrants.

Thanks are due to a number of people: to Maurice J. Martin, M.D. (ABMS President), whose leadership and commitment to board certification are manifest in his continuing strong support of these conferences; to the ABMS staff who are extraordinarily helpful as always; to J. Lee Dockery, M.D., executive vice president of ABMS without whom none of this could have happened; and to Philip G. Bashook, Ed.D. who is the staff person for COSEP and in that role has made important contributions in both conceptualizing and implementing the conference program.

I would also like to thank the members of COSEP, all of whom have shared in conceiving the conference: George E. Cruft, M.D., Joel A. DeLisa, M.D., Stewart B. Dunsker, M.D., Francis P. Hughes, Ph.D., Edward A. Krull, M.D., Charles L. Puckett, M.D., Mary Ann Reinhart, Ph.D., and Fred G. Smith, M.D.

A special thanks is due the ABMS staff who produced these proceedings: Gail Strejc for her work in type-setting the manuscript for desk-top publishing, Alexis Rodgers for guiding the publication process, and Marci Burr, Bobbye Higdon, Evalyn Moore, and Kathleen Hoinacki for their secretarial efforts.

Elliott L. Mancall, M.D.
Chairman, ABMS Committee on Study of Evaluation Procedures
Co-Editor

PART 1

THE ORAL EXAMINATION: AN HISTORICAL PERSPECTIVE

The Oral Examination: An Historical Perspective

Elliott L. Mancall, M.D.
Hahnemann University/Medical College of Pennsylvania

The issue of the oral examination as part of the board certification process has long attracted the attention of the American Board of Medical Specialties (ABMS). Two major conferences have been devoted to this matter—in 1975 and again in 1982—but, in fact, threads of controversy can be traced back through many years of discussions and round tables, and continue in one form or another to the present day; indeed, this 1995 conference on the oral examination is itself testimony to the enduring interest in this examining technique on the part of the now twenty-four ABMS Member Boards.

The perceived contributions of this examining tool have been described on a number of occasions. Linn,[1] for example, stresses the ability of the oral examination to measure behavioral aspects of a candidate's practice beyond cognition alone; to provide interaction with gender and ethnicity; to generate anxiety; to relate to clinical skills and personality; and to provide a bridge between cognitive and behavioral evaluations. Rosinski[2] emphasizes three qualities for which the oral exam was often considered particularly well suited: evaluation of the candidate's fund of knowledge, his (or her) capacity for problem solving, and his (or her) personal characteristics, i.e., noncognitive attributes such as response to stress, the ability to react quickly to changing circumstances, the ability to express ideas, and personal attitudes.

With Rosinski,[2] most today would agree that the first of these, i.e., evaluations of a candidate's knowledge base, can be carried out more effectively with other testing techniques. There is some disagreement as to whether problem-solving capability can be more efficiently appraised by other means. It is, however, the necessity of assessing noncognitive elements of clinical performance that remains, for many, the single most important reason for including the oral examination in the certification process.

In this vein, Abrahamson[3] has enumerated a series of candidate attributes which require direct observation of, and interaction between, the candidate and the examiner:

(1) Interpersonal skills;
(2) The ability to readjust, to respond to a new problem or challenge;
(3) The ability to respond to changing situations; and
(4) The ability to assume an appropriate role and perform accordingly, thus demonstrating acceptability to the specialty and in turn implying possession of a suitable professional demeanor and attitude.

Finally, quoting Perlmutter[4] at the 1983 ABMS conference, ". . . oral examinations should be able to test something more than a written examination, that is, the ability of the candidate to assimilate and integrate information, to make management decisions, and to think on his or her feet." Abrahamson[3] among many others concludes that it is only through the vehicle of the oral exam that such candidate qualities can suitably be assessed.

Despite the foregoing, there is wide agreement that the oral examination possesses inherent difficulties that cannot be ignored.[5] Problems with using the oral examination are of sufficient magnitude to some observers to negate the presumed advantages of the technique, and in fact have long been recognized. In brief,[3] these problems are: objectivity, reliability, validity, and cost. Will different scorers arrive at the same score? Will repeated measurements provide consistent responses? Does the examination measure what it sets out to do? Is it cost effective? Many of these issues can be addressed, as Perlmutter[4] has emphasized, by rigorous standardization applied not only to the contents of the examination itself, but also to the examiners (necessitating, for example, a program of examiner training) and to the grading system. Finberg and Lloyd,[6] in summarizing the 1983 conference, present a series of suggested guidelines for an ideal oral examination which incorporate and extend these notions.

It is inevitable that many of these views, both pro and con, will surface during today's conference, quite possibly in contexts far removed from medicine and the specialty movement. No further comment would be appropriate or useful, therefore, in these introductory remarks.

It would be helpful at this point, however, and as background to this conference, to review where we are presently in terms of usage of the oral examination, and how we got there. While recognizing the continuing controversy about the ultimate value and role of the oral examination in certification, and in the face of unanswered questions about costs in an increasingly cost-sensitive environment, it remains nonetheless true that currently 15 of the 24 ABMS Member Boards do in fact continue to utilize this form of examination as a vital part of the process of evaluation for initial certification. Since the American Board of Radiology (ABR) and the American Board of Psychiatry and Neurology (ABPN) each administer two distinct examinations—the former in diagnostic radiology and radiation oncology, the latter in psychiatry and neurology—the total of oral exams is actually 17. It is only ABPN, incidentally, which continues to use live patients as a significant part of the examination format.

Historically, from with the foundation of the organized specialty board movement in 1917 through 1950, all boards utilized oral examinations, generally with live patients (Table 1). In fact, prior to 1950 written examinations (primarily of the essay type) were considered less reliable than the oral technique. In the 1950s and later, however, basically following the lead of the National Board of Medical Examiners (NBME), the value of the oral examination was increasingly called into question. The American Board of Family Practice (ABFP), the American Board of Allergy and Immunology (ABA/I), the American Board of Nuclear Medicine (ABNM), and the American Board of Medical Genetics (ABMG), all established since the late 1960s, have never pursued the oral examination option, and oral examinations were discarded by a number of older boards; the largest defections, precipitated mostly by logistic issues, were those of the American Board of Internal Medicine (ABIM) in 1970 and the American Board of Pediatrics (ABPeds) in 1989. Interestingly, and perhaps paradoxically in the face of this apparent trend, the American Board of Emergency Medicine (ABEM), approved as a primary board in 1979, has used oral examinations from the outset.

Table 1. Evolution of the Oral Examination

1917-1950	All boards use oral exams
1950-1970	Oral exams dropped by
	Dermatology (1975)
	Pathology (1958)
	Preventive Medicine (1969)
1969	Family Practice approved; no oral exam
1970	Oral exam dropped by Internal Medicine Cardiovascular (1974)
1971	Nuclear Medicine approved; no oral exam
1971	Allergy and Immunology approved; no oral exam
1979	Emergency Medicine approved; using oral exam
1989	Oral exam dropped by Pediatrics
1991	Medical Genetics approved; no oral exam
1995	Fifteen boards using oral exam

Of the 15 boards currently administering oral examinations, none presently have plans to eliminate this form of assessment. All also utilize written examinations as a qualifying examination; achieving a passing grade in the written is a prerequisite for sitting for the oral certifying component.

A survey of current usage among these 15 boards indicates that there is no universal format for the oral examination. Four principle modes can be identified:

1. Long cases (20 minutes or more)
2. Live patients (American Board of Psychiatry & Neurology)
3. Written vignettes
4. Chart stimulated recall and interviews (American Boards of Emergency Medicine, Obstetrics and Gynecology, and Orthopaedic Surgery)

A number of boards utilize supplemental material such as slides, radiographs and other images, and videotaped patient encounters.

Based on contemporary practice,[7] the characteristics of a standardized oral examination may be summarized as follows:

Table 2. Standardized Oral Examination

1. Duration: 2.3 hours (+/- 1 hour)
2. Number of sessions: 3.9 (+/- 2.3)
3. Number of examiners per session: 1 - 2
4. Number of cases/session: 4.8 (+/- 2.2)
5. Session duration: 33 minutes (+/- 10.8 minutes)

All boards have examiner training programs, formal orientation sessions for new examiners lasting from two hours to a half-day or more. All boards evaluate the examiners as well. Scoring is carried out differently among the various boards. Each candidate is scored after each case encounter separately and independently by each examiner, but the format for scoring varies. Two boards use only pass/fail categories while eight also include conditional grades (at times with added nuances of high or low condition). Numerical rating scales are used in seven examinations. Discrepancies in scores from session to session, i.e., mixed passing and failing scores, are resolved in discussions among the examiners and/or directors. Overall passing rates for the 1994 examination range between 65 percent and 80 percent; for first-time takers the range was 72 percent to 91 percent. All boards of course document candidate performance, such documentation being especially important in instances of candidate failure.

One may conclude then that the oral examination as a component in the specialty certifying process remains very much alive and at least reasonably well. Experience over many years has permitted fine tuning not only of the contents of the examination itself but of the methodologies and apparatus of the total process. The work of refinement is however ongoing. All boards have regular programs of surveillance and reevaluation so as to maintain the oral and, of course, the entire certifying process as a fair, credible and cost-effective product.

References

1. Linn BS. Unique contributions of oral examinations. In *Oral Examinations in Medical Specialty Board Certification,* Lloyd JS, Ed., American Board of Medical Specialties, Evanston, IL, 1983; pp. 13-16.

2. Rosinski EF. The oral examination as an educational assessments procedure. In *Evaluating the Skills of Medical Specialists,* Lloyd JS and Langsley DG, Eds., American Board of Medical Specialties, Evanston, IL, 1976; pp. 101-104.

3. Abrahamson S. The oral examination: the case for and the case against. In *Evaluating the Skills of Medical Specialists,* Lloyd JS and Langsley DG, Eds., American Board of Medical Specialties, Evanston, IL, 1976; pp. 121-124.

4. Perlmutter AD. Standardization of oral examinations. In *Oral Examinations in Medical Specialty Board Certification,* Lloyd JS, Ed., American Board of Medical Specialties, Evanston, IL, 1983; pp. 63-65.

5. McGuire C. Studies of the oral examination: experience with orthopedic surgery. In *Evaluating the Skills of Medical Specialists,* Lloyd JS and Langsley DG, Eds., American Board of Medical Specialties, Evanston, IL, 1976; pp. 105-109.

6. Finberg L and Lloyd JS. Suggested guidelines for ideal oral examinations. In *Oral Examinations in Medical Specialty Board Certification,* Lloyd JS, Ed., American Board of Medical Specialties, Evanston, IL, 1983; pp. 125-130.

7. American Board of Medical Specialties, unpublished survey of Member Boards, January, 1995.

PART 2

ASSESSING REASONING AND JUDGMENT

Assessing Reasoning and Judgment

Gordon G. Page, Ed.D.
Faculty of Medicine
University of British Columbia

It is a privilege to address you this morning on the topic of "Assessing Reasoning and Judgment." From a selfish perspective I see this next 30 minutes as an opportunity to convey several messages that I feel are of great importance to the process of certifying medical competence. My task of course is to convince you of the importance of my views.

I believe that the assessment of competence is a greater challenge in medicine than in most other educational arenas. The conceptual processes required to resolve often ill defined problems are exceedingly complex, and the topics that I will address today—reasoning and judgment—are central elements of these complex processes. I am admittedly also biased in believing that relative to other educational arenas, medicine is at the forefront in the assessment of competence. The ABMS Member Boards have contributed to this leadership position through, in some instances, forty to fifty years of ongoing development of the certification examination programs. The American Board of Medical Specialties itself has contributed through convening meetings such as this, and by publishing the conference proceedings. These ABMS publications convey the wisdom of past and present contributors to the area of competency assessment in medicine; some of you are here today.

It was an interesting exercise to review the proceedings of previous conferences in an attempt to identify what I might contribute to today's deliberations that would build upon these conferences. Considerable attention has already been given to the following issues which are of fundamental importance in discussing the assessment of reasoning and judgment.

1. **Case Specificity.** This phrase was coined to describe the fact that a candidate's performance in resolving one clinical case is a poor predictor of performance on other cases, and that to generalize about a candidate's level of performance requires testing that candidate on many cases.[1]
2. **Reliability.** This issue relates primarily to the need to *sample adequately* across the domain of clinical problems for which the candidate is accountable. Case specificity of performance requires a large sample to obtain acceptable reliability for the overall exam.
3. **Content Validity.** This issue relates to the need to obtain a *representative sample* across the domain of problems for which the candidate is accountable, and the need to use *examination blueprints* to guide the selection of examination content. Content validity and reliability are preconditions for drawing correct inferences from an examination score to a candidate's general level of competence, and such inferences are the goal of any certification process.
4. **Training Examiners and Standardizing Cases in Oral Examinations.** It has been common practice in standardizing oral exams to train examiners and standardize cases across exam sessions. I would anticipate those in the audience using oral exams for certification have been doing this since the mid-1970s.

I will assume that current examination processes address those issues appropriate for certification examinations, and my task is to build upon this foundation. I will pose two fundamental questions about the assessment of reasoning and judgment, and then answer each question from what I hope will be new perspectives.

You are encouraged to look closely at *what* you measure, that is:

> "What questions should you ask in assessing candidates' clinical reasoning and judgment skills?"

and *how* you measure, that is:

> "What techniques should you use?"

All 24 Boards use multiple-choice questions (MCQs) for their written examinations, and in addition 15 Boards use an oral examination. The perspective on *what* to measure pertains both to written and oral examinations, and is based upon recent work in cognitive psychology on medical expertise. In addressing the issue of *how* to measure judgment and reasoning, I will challenge the reliance on multiple-choice questions (MCQs). This challenge is based upon a review of some widely cited, but I believe misinterpreted, data about the relationship of performance on multiple-choice questions to expertise in clinical reasoning and judgment. This challenge will also cite studies recently conducted at the Medical Council of Canada on the short answer question format. The goal, therefore, is twofold: (1) to provide guidelines for what to assess in judging candidates' clinical reasoning and judgment, and (2) to encourage questioning the current commitment to the MCQ as the sole form of written test item to be used in a certification examination.

What to Assess

First let's look at what to assess. My home is in beautiful Vancouver (where it rains on the odd occasion) at the University of British Columbia Medical School (UBC). UBC holds the distinction of having the last traditional medical curriculum in Canada, and this presentation will follow tradition by starting with the fundamentals—the basic sciences if you wish.

At the outset, agreement is needed on the meaning of some terms. Several different interrelated terms are used to describe the thought processes a physician uses in diagnosing and managing a clinical problem. The terms are: *reasoning, problem solving, judgment,* and *decision making.* Much of the literature on evaluating clinical competence uses these terms somewhat interchangeably. For purposes of clarity, the terms *problem solving* and *judgment* will not be used here, and meanings stipulated for *reasoning* and *decision making*. These definitions may fly in the face of how terms are used currently, but they will provide a common language for discussion.

Clinical Reasoning

Clinical reasoning is the physician's thought process. Research on the thinking of physicians has suggested that this thought process is often hypothetico-deductive reasoning,[2] characterized by: (1) the generation of hypotheses about a patient's problem, and (2) gathering and interpreting data to rule out or support these hypotheses. Effective clinical reasoning, however, is not always a hypothetico-deductive process. For a highly skilled physician, for example, it may more closely resemble a pattern recognition process with some patient cases. The chart stimulated recall process used by some boards is one effective way of uncovering a physician's reasoning. How a physician reasons through a problem can be unraveled to some extent by asking questions such as, "Why did you order that investigation?", or "What do this patient's blood values mean to you?", or "What suggested to you that this patient may have cellulitis?" An initial recommendation is that questions like these, which assess clinical reasoning or thought processes, are not the type of questions to use in a certifying examination, for neither oral nor written components.

Clinical Decisions

The thought processes of clinical reasoning culminate in clinical decisions that can be "observed" as the physician's clinical actions. Clinical decisions most commonly refer to a patient's diagnoses and treatment. More generally, clinical decisions are the basis of all actions taken by a physician in the work-up and management of a patient. Clinical decisions underlie specific history questions, or the ordering of a specific investigation. All of these clinical actions—identifying diagnoses, selecting treatments, asking questions, ordering investigations—are observable behaviors. Observing the actions on written and oral examinations provides the basis for assessing the physician's clinical decision making. A second recommendation is that an assessment of the clinical decisions relative to the key steps in resolving a patient's problem should be emphasized in both the written and oral components of certifying examinations. This recommendation, of course, implies that the title of this presentation should be changed from "Assessing Reasoning and Judgment" to "Assessing Clinical Decision Making." To summarize, clinical reasoning is a thought process leading to clinical decisions; examination questions should focus on the decisions and not on the reasoning.

Georges Bordage and his colleagues[3,4] have developed a conceptual model of physicians' knowledge structures and clinical reasoning which provides a rationale for this suggestion. Bordage's model is based upon studies of how medical students and physicians in practice analyze clinical problems. In this model, four types of knowledge and reasoning are identified: *reduced, dispersed, elaborated,* and *compiled.*

Reduced Knowledge

When presented with a clinical problem, a physician with reduced knowledge simply does not possess the knowledge needed to understand and resolve the problem.

Dispersed Knowledge

A physician with dispersed knowledge may possess the knowledge, but it is memorized as unrelated lists such that its relevance to the problem at hand is not seen.

Elaborated Knowledge

A physician with elaborated knowledge possesses the necessary knowledge, sees its relevance to the problem, and through logical reasoning applies the knowledge to the resolution of the problem.

Compiled Knowledge

The physician with compiled knowledge has had prior experience with the problem, does not need to engage in a detailed reasoning process and, perhaps more through pattern recognition, is concise and focused in resolving the problem.

Physicians with elaborated and compiled knowledge are competent at making good clinical decisions, whereas those with reduced and dispersed knowledge are not. To illustrate these four levels of knowledge and reasoning, here are examples of four physicians' responses to the same patient case presenting with a neurological problem. (Figure 1)

Figure 1. Patient with Neurological Problem

Mr. B., a 63-year-old longshoreman, complains that he has had numbness in the right arm for the past three-to-four months, mainly in the hand and worse at night.

He smokes a pack-and-a-half of cigarettes a day and drinks rarely.

He noticed that his left hand has also been numb for the past two months or so, but to a lesser extent than on the right side. He has always been in excellent health. The rest of the history is unremarkable. The physical exam is also unremarkable except for some atrophy of the intrinsic muscles in the right hand with weakness of the abduction of the fingers as well as decreased sensitivity in the fourth and fifth fingers; slight muscular wasting in the left hand with no sensory problem; and an absent right brachioradialis reflex. At this point in the encounter the following signs are revealed: brisk reflexes in the lower limbs with a nonsustained clonus in both feet.

Looking at four physicians' responses to this case may remind some of residents they know.

Clinician R
(Reduced Knowledge): I don't know. I can't seem to remember what brisk reflexes and clonus mean. I'll just move on.

According to Bordage, Clinician R (Reduced Knowledge) can find no connection between his store of knowledge and the patient's findings, either because he cannot access the knowledge, or never acquired it to begin with. His response is largely one of inertia, and his knowledge and discourse are characterized as "reduced."

Clinician D
(Dispersed Knowledge): Yes, upper limbs, lower limbs. Yes. It looks like the extremities are involved. This could be alcoholism, Vitamin B_{12} deficiency, or polyneuritis.

Clinician D (Dispersed Knowledge) connects the patient's findings with ready-made, static lists of diagnoses, but does not challenge the diagnoses through reference to the findings. His reasoning is highly "dispersed," even though his knowledge base may be high.

Clinician E (Elaborated Knowledge): What we have here is an older man with a gradual onset of a motor and sensory problem that is bilateral yet asymmetrical. There is a peripheral motor involvement in the upper limbs as opposed to a pyramidal problem in the lower limbs. I can exclude a peripheral problem in the lower limbs. A central cause is likely ... with cervical arthrosis causing a myelopathy at C8-T1 as well as bilateral radiculopathies.

Clinician E (Elaborated Knowledge) sees the links between the patient's findings and the possible explanations for these findings, and uses "elaborated" networks of relationships in his memory and methodical reasoning to diagnose the patient's problem.

Clinician C (Compiled Knowledge): Here's an element that makes me think of a sublesional symptomatology secondary to a cervical myelopathy that would also give radiculopathies on both sides at C8. It's surprising that this patient is not complaining of cervical pain.

Clinician C (Compiled Knowledge) quickly recognizes a pattern that he has "compiled" in his memory pointing to specific causes, which evoke a search for neck pain that is a missing element in the pattern.

What specific guidance does the Bordage model provide for assessing physicians' ability to resolve clinical problems at the certification level? There are three main messages, two concerning what not to measure, and one identifying what should be measured.

1. The first message is that the assessment should not test a physician's knowledge base. Physicians with dispersed knowledge, those who have a mind plugged with memorized information, may do well to recall knowledge, but would not do well on test questions which require application of the same knowledge to resolve cases. A common principle in creating multiple-choice questions (MCQs) is that knowledge application, and not knowledge per se, should be tested. This principle can be applied readily if exam questions use cases that demand some form of clinical decision making. In 1904, Osler advised that no teaching should be done without a patient as a text.[5] The natural corollary is only evaluate with a patient as the context.

2. The second message from Bordage's work is that the assessment should not employ questions testing physicians' clinical reasoning. Questions which test the clinical reasoning processes (hypothesis generation, data acquisition and analysis) may penalize the real clinical expert; the physician operating at the compiled level of knowledge does not need to engage in a hypothetico-deductive process to resolve clinical problems.[3] This observation provides an explanation for the results of many past studies on the construct validity of case-based examinations like patient management problems or case-based orals. These studies typically compared medical students and residents at different levels of training with physicians who had been in practice for five to ten years, on the expectation that greater training and experience would lead to higher scores. A common finding was that practicing physicians obtained lower scores than some resident groups, largely because the scoring systems rewarded thoroughness of data gathering in which the experienced, "compiled," physician did not engage.
3. The third message is that the assessment should employ questions which concentrate on the key clinical decisions leading to the resolution of a clinical problem. The physician with compiled knowledge will quickly make these decisions, and the physician with elaborated knowledge will most likely get to them through a detailed reasoning process. In the Medical Council of Canada's recently completed project to develop a new examination of clinical decision making, the key clinical decisions for a problem were labeled the problem's "key features," and defined as the critical steps in the problem's resolution.[6,7] In this project, and in the American College of Physicians' most recent Medical Knowledge Self Assessment Program (MKSAP), test committees of physicians typically identified two-to-four key features for a problem. Key features are, of course, unique for each clinical problem.

The recommendation *to assess* key clinical decisions and *not assess* aspects of the clinical reasoning process applies to any form of examination question, but particularly relates to oral examination formats which use rating forms or, even worse, checklists. Checklists identify specific physician behaviors which often mirror the hypothetico-deductive process and reward thorough data gathering. Let me illustrate this point.

In Vancouver there is a program which presents practicing physicians with a series of standardized patients in a multi-station examination. A physician is given ten minutes with each standardized patient and five minutes to write progress notes on that patient. The physician is rated by the patient on a checklist of behaviors relating to history taking and/or physical examination, and the progress notes are marked for recording key findings, accuracy of diagnosis and appropriateness of a management plan. A physician is often observed to spend only three or four minutes of the allotted ten minutes with the patient. The checklist may reveal that the physician did no more than ask two or three questions of the 15 to 20 that were listed, and the mark derived from the checklist suggests that this physician has performed poorly. This physician's progress notes however may contain the key clinical findings, correctly identify the patient's problem or problems, and present a sound management plan. Such physicians likely possess compiled knowledge for the problem, but are penalized on the checklist because they do not engage in a hypothetico-deductive process. The progress notes offer a far better basis for judging competence in problem resolution than the checklists. The former records clinical decisions and actions, and the latter, checklists, pertains more to an imposed process of clinical reasoning. Checklists of data gathering behaviors do have their place in medical education, but a certifying examination is not one of those places; unless, the checklists are highly focused only upon the critical steps in the resolution of the patient's problem, the problem's key features.

Up to this point, the focus has been on what to assess when judging candidates' competence in resolving clinical problems. The main messages are that assessments should concentrate on the candidates' ability to make key clinical decisions, and not on steps in the clinical reasoning process, or on the requisite knowledge base.

How to Assess

To change direction, let us now look at the techniques used to assess clinical decision making. I will attempt to support what I believe may be an unpopular proposition regarding questions which present candidates with lists of options. The main target is the multiple-choice question (MCQ). Implicit in these remarks is support for written examination formats and for oral examinations which require candidates to *generate* clinical decisions in contrast to *selecting* them from lists of options. First, a logical argument, and then empirical data will be presented in support of the proposition that the specialty boards should reduce their reliance on MCQs in favor of question formats that require candidates to supply a response. This proposition is offered while fully recognizing that there are compelling arguments and approximately 50 years of satisfied users supporting MCQs. Most support for MCQs is based upon issues of cost and test score reliability. In contrast, the arguments against MCQs will focus largely on issues of validity—that is, do scores from examinations composed of multiple-choice questions provide the basis for correct inferences about candidates' clinical decision-making abilities?

The Logical Argument. In the mid-1970s, I had the pleasure of being one of two external reviewers of proposals to develop the certifying examination for the American Board of Emergency Medicine. Michigan State University's proposal, with Jack Maatsch as one of its principal architects, was selected to develop the examination. The key issue that separated the Michigan State proposal from others was the fidelity to reality of their proposed assessment methods. Their proposal suggested that the certification examination should adopt assessment procedures which replicate, as closely as possible, the challenges board candidates faced in their clinical roles. This concept of fidelity to reality was seen by Jack Maatsch to be essential to the validity of the assessment process.

In the context of our current discussion of clinical decision-making skills, the concept of fidelity is also of utmost importance. In real life, patient diagnoses are not selected from lists, nor are treatment decisions. Yet this is how MCQs test candidates' abilities to make correct diagnoses and select appropriate treatments. Applying the Bordage model, when a candidate possesses *elaborated* or *compiled* knowledge about a problem the list of options in a multiple-choice question may serve no useful purpose. The candidate would likely make the correct clinical decision without the list of options. For the candidate operating at the *dispersed level* of knowledge, the list can provide a major cuing effect. This seems ironic. It is these weaker candidates that the entire certification process is designed to identify. Questions which require candidates to generate their own clinical decisions provide a much higher fidelity to the real situation than selecting answers from lists within a multiple-choice question or other objective test formats. Intuitively, the argument presented against MCQs and other forms of questions to assess clinical decision making which present lists of options may seem convincing; but are there data to support the argument?

The Empirical Argument. Many studies have been conducted comparing scores on multiple-choice questions (MCQs) or true/false (T/F) examinations and examinations of the same content using short answer questions. The general finding is that the correlation between sets of scores from MCQ or T/F tests and short answer tests examining the same content is typically higher than 0.90 when the correlation is corrected for the lack of reliability of the two tests.[8-13] This result has been widely interpreted to mean that the two tests measure the same thing or, more accurately, two highly related things. With this result, and with a view to objectivity and reduced costs for grading tests, the MCQ test format has been recommended. In the context of a certification examination, it is worthwhile to look closely at the basis of this recommendation, the high correlation coefficient.

Table 1 presents a set of hypothetical but typical data from an MCQ examination and a short answer examination, each with 100 items testing the same content, with respective and generous reliabilities of 0.85 and 0.80.

Table 1. Examination Scores (%) and Relationships

	Scores										Means
Cand	1	2	3	4	5	6	7	8	9	10	
MCQ*	85	80	77	74	71	68	65	62	60	50	69
SA*	80	67	73	58	61	55	40	47	43	30	55
Diff	5	13	4	16	10	13	25	15	17	20	

No. of test items = 100 MCQ & SA observed corr. = .95

Reliabilities = .85 and .80 MCQ & SA corrected corr. = 1.00

*MCQ is multiple-choice question format; SA is short answer question format.

The observed correlation between these two sets of data is 0.95, and when this correlation is corrected for attenuation due to the lack of reliability of the two tests, the corrected correlation is 1.00. The corrected correlation of 1.00 indicates that, to the degree that these tests are reliably measuring some attribute, they seem to be measuring two attributes which are perfectly related. Looking closely at the two rows of data in Table 1, there are both similarities and differences. There is no doubt that the ranking of candidates is similar on both tests, but not identical. This is what the high observed correlation coefficient conveys, and the corrected correlation of 1.00 indicates that if you factor in the recognition that these tests are not perfectly reliable instruments, the rankings on the two tests would be identical. However, there are some major differences in these two distributions of scores.

The mean score on the short answer test is lower by 14 percent and, more importantly, there is a trend for the weaker candidates to perform at a considerably lower level on the short answer test. It is these people who benefit most from the cuing provided by the list of MCQ options, and from the fact that selecting an answer from the list of the five MCQ options provides a 20 percent success rate by chance alone (one chance in five they will guess the keyed answer). The reference to high correlation coefficients between MCQ and short answer tests to support the use of MCQs is highly misleading. The correlation coefficients hide the illustrated differences in score distributions, differences which are of critical importance in the context of certification examinations.

Not all correlational studies of MCQ and short answer examinations have produced high correlation coefficients similar to those just discussed. In 1978, Fredricksen and colleagues at the Educational Testing Service observed that the studies reporting these high correlations typically related scores from MCQ examinations *to* short answer adaptions of these MCQ examinations. They took the reverse tack in test development. From 1978 to 1981 they conducted a series of studies of equivalent MCQ tests developed *from* short answer tests. Their test items were designed to assess hypothesis generation and data gathering skills which they referred to as problem solving skills. They first developed short answer versions of their tests and from these developed parallel tests using multiple-choice questions to assess the same skills. The observed correlations of performance across the two test forms were less than 0.20. They concluded that at least for their problem-solving tests, the MCQ and short answer question formats did not measure the same set of cognitive skills, and that the MCQ questions appeared to be poor substitutes for the higher fidelity short answer questions.[14] This study lends further support to Jack Maatsch's position regarding the importance of fidelity in the assessment process.

Other studies of identical questions in MCQ and short answer formats have looked for format effects by analyzing differences in response distributions across the two formats. In this conference, Dr. Dale Dauphinee will report on the use of "key features" problems to assess clinical decision-making in the Medical Council of Canada's Qualifying Examination. Short answer questions are used in this examination. Georges Bordage and I were the investigators in the six-year study that led to the introduction of this examination. Part of our research focused on the differences in the response distributions to the same question presented in a short answer format and then with a menu of options.[6,7] Let us look at two questions from that examination, and the distribution of responses from the short answer and menu formats for these questions. On the examination, each question is presented in the context of a case.

Figure 2. Sample Question
Short Answer Format

What would you recommend for this patient?
List up to five recommendations.

1. ______________________________
2. ______________________________
3. ______________________________
4. ______________________________
5. ______________________________

Figure 2 is an example of a question presented in its short answer format; it requires candidates to write in their responses.

Figure 3. Sample Question Menu Format

What would you recommend for this patient?
Select up to five recommendations.

1. Amoxicillin for six days
2. Antacids
3. Beta blocker
4. Cholecystectomy
5. Diet to lose weight
6. Hiatus hernia repair
7. High fiber diet
8. Histamine-2 blocker
9. Laxative
10. Low fat diet
11. Nonsteroidal anti-inflammatory drug
12. Raise the head of the bed 15 cm
13. Sleep with extra pillow
14. Stool softener
15. Vagotomy and pyloroplasty

Figure 3 is the same question in its menu format. Candidates select their responses from the menu of options listed.

Table 2. Distribution of Responses (% Correct)

What would you recommend for this patient?
Select up to five recommendations.

	Short Answer	Menu
1. Amoxicillin for six days	0	0
2. Antacids	**24**	**70**
3. Beta blocker	0	2
4. Cholecystectomy	24	16
5. Diet to lose weight	**59**	**87**
6. Hiatus hernia repair	0	5
7. High fiber diet	1	34
8. Histamine-2 blocker	**17**	**31**
9. Laxative	0	1
10. Low fat diet	**34**	**63**
11. Nonsteroidal anti-inflammatory drug	0	1
12. Raise the head of the bed 15 cm	**58**	**82**
13. Sleep with extra pillow	3	31
14. Stool softener	0	3
15. Vagotomy and Pyloroplasty	0	0

Table 2 contains data on the distribution of responses to the question in each format—the percentage of candidates writing in or selecting each option. The numbers in bold identify the keyed "correct" answers to the question. Note that presenting a menu of options seems to make it much more likely that candidates will provide the correct responses.

Table 3. Distribution of Responses (% Correct)

In your initial treatment of this baby, what would you now order? Select up to four

	Short Answer	Menu
1. Acetylcysteine (Mucomyst) enema	0	0
2. Atropine	0	0
3. Discontinue oral feeding	**28**	**71**
4. Enema until clear	0	0
5. Gastric lavage	1	0
6. Intravenous fluids	**73**	**79**
7. Intravenous antibiotics	0	0
8. Lactose-free diet	2	6
9. Nasogastric suction	**28**	**52**
10. Pancreatic enzyme	1	0
11. Small feeding	8	8
12. Surgical consultation	**52**	**87**
13. Total parenteral nutrition	1	17
14. Tube feeding	0	6
15. Weigh daily	0	24

Table 3 is another question depicting the same pattern of response differences across the short answer and menu formats. The frequency of responses to the keyed items is generally much higher in the questions presenting a menu of options. The average score increased 20 percent from the short answer to the matched menu questions in these studies for the Medical Council of Canada.

It is hoped that the logical argument and this data challenging the use of test items with lists encourages further thinking and questioning about the commitment to MCQs to test clinical decision making. There are excellent opportunities, through research and development programs of boards, to review the relationships between MCQ exam results and the higher fidelity test formats obtained through short answer written questions, oral examinations, and perhaps other formats (e.g., standardized patient encounters and free response computer-based examinations). In investigating these relationships, dig beneath the often misleading correlational analyses commonly reported in the existing literature.

In response to the question posed by the title of this conference, "Assessing Clinical Reasoning: If not the Oral Examination, What?," the key feature question format, when presented in the context of cases, including its flexibility in formats and answer keys, provides an appealing alternative to oral examinations for examining some important clinical skills.

Summary

In relationship to current methods of assessing clinical reasoning and judgment in certification programs, this presentation attempted to provide guidelines on "what to assess" and "how to assess." The guidelines and comments are built upon the issue of test validity which is fundamental to any testing — that is, are the test scores from the certifying examinations providing the basis for correct inferences about candidates' clinical competence?

In answering the question of what to measure in a certification examination, the emphasis should be on the assessment of key clinical decisions, and not on processes of clinical reasoning. The rationale for this suggestion is grounded in studies of clinical expertise which demonstrate that expert clinicians with *compiled* knowledge often arrive at correct clinical decisions and effectively resolve problems without engaging in a hypothetico-deductive reasoning process involving extensive hypothesis generation and data gathering. Further, it is suggested that the assessment process should not measure the requisite knowledge a candidate must possess, because such assessments may not identify candidates whose knowledge is present but dispersed, and who may be unable to use the knowledge in an elaborated or compiled way in resolving clinical problems.

How to measure clinical decision making is discussed beginning with a logical argument and data to support the proposition that: the extensive reliance on the multiple-choice question format for certification examinations poses a threat to the validity of judgments about the weaker candidates. You are encouraged to investigate this issue further and consider short answer questions and other question formats which provide a higher fidelity when measuring important thought processes in clinical medicine. The recommendations offered in this presentation are important to the validity of any certification process and it is hoped they will be kept in mind while considering the other papers in this conference.

References

1. Norman G, et al. A Review of Recent Innovations in Assessment. In *Directions in Clinical Assessment. Report of the First Cambridge Conference on the Assessment of Clinical Competence,* Wakeford, R, (Ed.) (pp. 8-27). Cambridge, England: Office of the Regius Professor of Physic, Cambridge University School of Clinical Medicine, Addenbrooke's Hospital, Cambridge, England, 1985.

2. Elstein A, Shulman L, Sprafka S. *Medical Problem Solving: An analysis of clinical reasoning.* Cambridge, Mass: Harvard University Press, 1978.

3. Bordage G. Elaborated Knowledge: A key to successful diagnostic thinking. *Acad Med;* 1994; 69:11:883-5.

4. Bordage G, Lemieux M. Semantic Structures and Diagnostic Thinking of Experts and Novices. *Acad Med;* 1991; 66:Supplement S70-2.

5. Osler W. On the Need of a Radical Reform in our Methods of Teaching Medical Students. *Med News;* 1904; 82:49-53.

6. Page G, Bordage G. The Medical Council of Canada's Key Features Project: A more valid written examination of clinical decision-making skills. *Acad Med* 1995; 70(2):104-10.

7. Page G, Bordage G, Allen T. Developing key feature problems and examinations to assess clinical decision-making skills. *Acad Med;* 1995; 70(3):194-201.

8. Patterson D. Do New and Old Type Examinations Measure Different Mental Functions? *School Society,* 1926; 24:246-8.

9. Bracht G, Hopkins K. The Commonality of Essay and Objective Tests of Academic Achievement. *Educ and Psychol Meas;* 1970; 30:359-64.

10. Crombag H. Comparison Between an Open-question Examination and a Multiple-choice Test. *Netherlands Tydschrift voor de Psychologie en haar Grensgebieden;* 1970; 25:349-59.

11. Norman G, Smith E, Powles A, Rooney P, et al. Factors Underlying Performance on Written Tests of Knowledge. *Med Educ;* 1987; 2:297-304.

12. Stalenhoef-Halling B, van der Vleuten C, Jaspers T, Fiolet T. The Feasibility, Acceptability and Reliability of Open-ended Questions in a Problem-based Learning Curriculum. In *Teaching and Assessing Clinical Competence,* Bender W, Hiemstra R, Scherpbier A, Swierstra R (Eds) Groningen: Boek Werk Publications, 1990, pp 552-557.

13. Schuwirth L, van der Vleuten C, Donkers H. The Use of Open-ended and Objective Questions: Cueing effects and precision of computer-based scoring. In *Gezond Onderwijs I,* van der Vleuten C, Scherpbier A, Pollemans M (Eds) Houten: Bohn, Stafleu, Van Loghum, 1992, 312-318.

14. Frederiksen N, Ward W, Case S, Carlson S, et al. *Development of Methods for Selection and Evaluation in Undergraduate Medical Education.* (ETS RR 81-4). Princeton, NJ: Educational Testing Service, 1981.

PART 3

POTENTIAL VALUE OF THE STANDARDIZED ORAL EXAMINATION

Advantages to Using the Oral Examination

Disadvantages to Using the Oral Examination

Discussion

Advantages to Using the Oral Examination

Mary Ann Reinhart, Ph.D.
American Board of Emergency Medicine

All certification decisions are based on judgment. The question is not whether a certifying body will utilize expert judgment, but rather, when and how will expert judgment be utilized in the development, administration, and scoring of its certification examinations?

Decisions about when and how to utilize expert judgment are closely tied to the method(s) used to evaluate certification candidates. Many here are familiar with a number of those methods, and several of the best methods will be discussed here today. These methods include written examinations, oral examination simulations, computer-administered knowledge examinations, computer simulations, standardized patients, and written key features examinations. Each of these methods can be reliable and valid for certain purposes. Our goal today is to explore which of these methods can be used to assess clinical reasoning for medical specialty certification.

Clinical reasoning is assessed by exploring a candidate's thinking or by investigating the outcomes of the candidate's reasoning. Evaluation of a candidate's reasoning and the outcomes of that reasoning can be captured by well-trained judges acting as oral examiners. I propose that this type of rich information, gathered and evaluated by oral examiners, is first, distinct from information about a person's degree of knowledge; second, cannot be captured by a written examination; and third, is most efficiently and inexpensively gathered and evaluated, in at least some medical specialties, by well-trained examiners assessing performance on standardized clinical simulations.

Three Types of Intelligence: General, Academic, and Practical

The distinct value of the type of information which can be gathered in oral examinations is supported by research from a number of measurement psychologists who are actively involved in the measurement and prediction of professional performance. These investigators[1,2,3,4] make a distinction among three types of intelligence which predict performance: **general intelligence**, **academic intelligence**, and **practical intelligence.**

1. They support the notion of a **general intelligence** factor which predicts professional performance across a broad range. This general intelligence factor is what is typically measured on an IQ test and is probably measured in the Medical College Admissions Test (MCAT).
2. **Academic intelligence** consists of content and rules that are formal and known by anyone who is interested and has the ability to pursue them. It is taught and valued in formal educational settings; and, in a medical specialty setting, it is the content of the medical specialty area. It is what is measured in most written examinations.
3. **Practical intelligence** is informal; it is knowledge about a professional area, rather than knowledge of the content of the area. It is learned by observation and modeling. In a medical specialty setting, a primary component of practical intelligence would be clinical reasoning and the clinical performance outcomes of that reasoning. It is measured best in simulations of practical, work-related situations.

In this schema of intelligence, each of these types of intelligence contributes to successful performance. Accordingly, the best prediction of successful performance would be based on the measurement of each of the three components of intelligence: general, academic, and practical. Specifically, the schema states that medical specialty performance would be measured best by having all candidates demonstrate at least adequate performance on independent measurements of general, academic, and practical intelligence.

American Board of Medical Specialties (ABMS) specialty boards do not measure general intelligence, but instead delegate this obligation to the medical schools, which require that applicants meet defined standards on the MCAT. The specialty certifying boards expect that all candidates have successfully demonstrated at least adequate general intelligence during their medical training.

On the other hand, most ABMS Member Boards do seek to measure both academic and practical intelligence, although these terms are not used as such. Typically boards seek to measure academic intelligence, or the content of the medical specialty, using either written or computer-administered comprehensive knowledge examinations. The boards seek to measure practical intelligence, including clinical reasoning and the outcomes of clinical reasoning as demonstrated in components of clinical performance, using a variety of methods. As an example, the American Board of Emergency Medicine (ABEM) uses a standardized oral examination based on simulations of actual emergency department cases for this purpose.

ABEM's experiences with its written and oral examinations support a theory of intelligence that states both academic and practical intelligence predict emergency department performance. Academic intelligence, as measured by the written examination, and practical intelligence, as measured by the oral examination, contribute unique information about a candidate's capabilities in Emergency Medicine. Findings from three major research studies conducted by ABEM over a period of 15 years support this theory of intelligence and reinforce the value of the ABEM oral examination in assessing practical intelligence.

ABEM Certification Examination Format

ABEM's certification examinations include a qualifying written comprehensive examination and a standardized oral examination based on simulations of emergency department cases administered by well-trained examiners who explore the candidate's reasoning and judge the candidate's performance.

The ABEM oral examination format has three distinct advantages over written and computer examination formats as a measure of practical intelligence. First, examiners in the oral examination can obtain the richness and complexity of performance information which is tied to clinical reasoning, is impossible to gather in a written examination format, and is expensive and difficult to gather in a computer format. Second, the performance information obtained in an oral examination format includes assessment of the practical knowledge, skills, and abilities needed in a day-to-day clinical setting, including information about clinical reasoning. Third, well-trained examiners can use a standardized scoring format to integrate the rich information obtained from candidates in an efficient, cost-effective, reliable, and valid manner. The performance ratings by independent examiners on the same candidate can be summed easily into an overall examination score.

The ABEM format is based on high fidelity simulations of actual emergency department cases. Cases are chosen on the basis of content, complexity, and level of difficulty. Real emergency medicine patient cases are selected and reformatted into the exam structure. Three or more critical incidents in each case are identified to guide case administration and scoring. Critical incidents are defined as those actions by the emergency department physician which must be completed successfully in order to manage a patient appropriately. Each critical incident is described in detail and linked with a specific performance rating. For example, timely administration of three sequential shocks to treat ventricular fibrillation in a patient experiencing a myocardial infarction would be assessed in the candidate's rating in patient management. The candidate would have to shock the patient according to defined guidelines developed by the board in order to receive an acceptable performance rating for patient management in the case.

In this format, candidates are presented with seven patient case situations, each administered by a different examiner. A total of 11 cases are administered to each candidate including one case undergoing field-testing. Each new case is field tested in order to collect data on the validity of the case administration procedures, to determine the case difficulty, and to determine the ability of the case to discriminate among identified groups of candidates. Field-test cases are not included in the candidate's examination score. The candidate's examination score is based upon the average performance ratings across six case situations which include ten cases.

Examiners are organized into teams, each managed by a team leader. Team leaders help train examiners and verify their performance. Chief examiners, who are directors of the board, review all performance ratings and examiner notes. Team leaders and chief examiners discuss administration or rating errors with the examiner, but examiners make the final scoring decisions on the cases they administer.

Examiners undergo six hours of rigorous training on case administration and scoring. They meet with the members of their teams for an additional three hours to discuss, practice, and demonstrate appropriate administration and scoring of the case simulations they will administer. Examiners themselves are monitored and evaluated on 17 criteria at each examination (See Figure 1).

Figure 1. Oral Examiner Performance Criteria (1995)

Candidate and Case Management
- Established a comfortable tone of interaction with candidates
- Started cases on time
- Maintained control of case timing
- Finished cases on time
- Introduced cases according to ABEM guidelines
- Managed case materials appropriately
- Administered cases according to agreed upon standards
- Played roles appropriately
- Cued appropriately
- Took comprehensive and readable notes

Case Scoring
- Demonstrated an understanding of the performance ratings
- Demonstrated an understanding of general scoring guidelines
- Demonstrated an understanding of the rating scale
- Scored cases according to specific ABEM case guidelines

Team Participation
- Demonstrated an acceptance of constructive criticism
- Participated positively in team meeting discussions
- Was on time for meetings during the week

Overall Team Leader Recommendation
- Retain for future examinations
- Suggested team assignment
- Consider for future team leader position

Problem areas in exam administration are discussed with the examiners, and examiners are expected to correct these faults. Those examiners who continue to have problems adhering to the board's administration and scoring guidelines are replaced.

Field testing cases, examination standardization, including the use of critical incidents, and rigorous examiner training and evaluation are the central components of the examination method.

Reliability and Validity of the ABEM Oral Examination

The ABEM examination was developed and assessed in 1979-1980,[5] and a predictive validity study was conducted in 1981-1983.[6] The unique contributions of the oral exam to the certification decision were described and investigated in a 1991-1993 study.[7] Each of these three major studies was planned in conjunction with ABEM and conducted by faculty at Michigan State University. Jack L. Maatsch, Ph.D., conducted the first two research projects; and John R. Hollenbeck, Ph.D., conducted the third.

The oral examination was developed and assessed in a two-year study of the examination. The examination was evaluated in 1979 in a field trial, and the examination was administered in 1980 for candidate certification.[5] Fourth-year medical students, second-year Emergency Medicine residents, and practice-eligible and residency-eligible candidates participated in the field trials. Reliability statistics for the examination included inter-rater [examiner] reliabilities of 0.79 and 0.82; within-case reliabilities of 0.97 and 0.96; and across-case reliabilities of 0.57.

The concurrent validity of the oral examination was demonstrated by correlating the field-test candidates' performances on the written knowledge examination with their performances on the oral examination. A correlation of 0.75 demonstrated that the two tests assess related, but not identical, knowledge, skills, and abilities.

The relationship between candidates' performances on the written and oral examinations was investigated further using LISREL (Linear Structural Relationships by the Method of Maximum Likelihood). The best fitting structural relationship describing what is measured by the ABEM examinations is a two-factor model in which the written and oral examinations measure both common and unique information. These findings support the view that the oral examination measures unique information beyond that measured in the written examination, as predicted by the theory of intelligence described earlier.

Predictive Validity Study

In 1981-1983, a predictive validity study of the oral examination was conducted with 246 certified emergency physicians.[6] The primary research question posed was "Does the oral examination predict actual performance on the diplomate's own emergency department cases?" A standardized method was developed to assess emergency physicians' performances based on their own patient charts. During the examination, the examiner conducts a structured interview based on patient charts in which the physician is asked about his or her performance when treating individual patients seen in the emergency department. This method was later refined into the "chart stimulated recall" oral examination and used as part of the board's original recertification examination program.[8]

Predictive validity as measured by the correlation between oral examination performance and chart stimulated recall performance was 0.45, using a full range of emergency physician ability. Emergency department performance accounted for almost twice the amount of variability in oral examination performance as it did for written examination performance. That is, performance on the oral examination was more strongly associated with performance in the emergency department than was the written examination performance.

Overall, these two studies indicated the oral examination is valid, and that it measures some components of Emergency Medicine performance which are distinct from those measured by the written examination.

The exact nature of the performance elements in emergency medical practice measured by the oral examination was not known at the time of these studies. An investigation of the unique information contributed by the oral examination was initiated by the board in 1990-1993. By 1990, the certification examinations had been given for 10 years, and the board felt it was important to investigate further the oral examination, and to reassess its value in the certification process.

ABEM posited two primary research questions:

1. "What is measured by the oral examination?"
2. "Which of the factors measured in the oral examination contribute unique information to the certification outcome after the information gathered by the written examination has been controlled?"

A prospective study[7] was conducted using data from all candidates who were examined in four sessions of the oral exam (n=236). Verbatim transcripts (n=314) of two oral examination cases were analyzed by examiner team leaders and nonphysician researchers. Based on this analysis, 11 new performance areas were defined (Figure 2).

Figure 2. Defined Performance Areas in the Oral Examination from Research Project (1991-1993)

Performance Area	Scale Anchor*	Scale Anchor
Pace and Expedience	Acts too slowly or quickly	Acts at an adequate pace
Decisiveness	Immobilized by indecision	Acts decisively
Clarity in Staff Orders	Orders are ambiguous or vague	Orders are clear and specific
Summarizing to Medical Staff	Provides incomplete summary of case to colleagues	Provides a complete summary of case to colleagues
Projects Emotional Control	Appears to panic on occasion	Constantly maintains composure
Consults Effectively	Asks for premature or inappropriate consultation	Consults appropriately in terms of time, issue and person
Efficiency of Ancillary Testing	Orders many inappropriate tests or procedures	Orders only appropriate tests or procedures
Foresight	Fails to anticipate future case developments	Anticipates all future case developments
Examiner's Presentation Accuracy	Provides misleading or inaccurate information	Provides relevant and accurate information
Examiner's Cuing	Hints at or divulges critical actions	Provides information judiciously
Examiner's Case Management	Mismanages pace or logical sequencing of case	Effectively controls pace and logical sequencing of case

*Scale anchors for three-point scale.

All of the candidates' written and oral examination performance outcomes were analyzed in order to determine the rating reliabilities and the distinct factors which were present. Our reliability analyses confirmed the strong interrater and within-case reliabilities previously observed.

We used factor analysis to study the candidates' scores on the eight oral exam performance ratings, their scores on the eleven performance ratings defined from case transcript analyses of the two cases, and their scores from written examinations. Six factors emerged from these analyses: The existing eight performance ratings formed one factor, the eleven new ratings formed four factors which are distinctly different from existing ratings, and the written examination formed a factor distinct from the others. The combined factors in the factor analysis accounted for 64 percent of the variability in the candidates' overall performance scores with the written examination accounting for eight percent, and the oral examination accounting for the remaining 56 percent of variability. The results clearly show that the oral examination measures performance areas which are not measured in the written examination.

It was also apparent from the analysis that the two oral examination cases yield unique information about clinical competence, composure when managing a patient, ability to solicit clinical data, and use of consultants in an effective manner. Clinical competence is measured by ratings on data acquisition, patient management, problem solving, patient outcome, resource utilization, interpersonal relations, and comprehension of pathophysiology. Composure is measured by ratings on pace and degree of expedience, decisiveness, and ability to project emotional control.

The final step in the study was to determine how much each of the factors contributed to the candidate's certification outcome (certified or not certified). A multiple regression analysis was used to assess the relative contributions of each of the factors described above, including the written examination performance, and the candidates' performances on the critical incidents. An equation with seven independent variables was produced.

The regression analyses show that candidates' performances on the two oral examinations used in the research contribute eight percent additional information for certification outcomes decisions beyond that obtained by the written examination which added fifteen percent. Again this supports the theory of intelligence described earlier. The majority of the additional information contributed by the candidates' performances on the two oral examinations was from initial performances (additions of five percent and eight percent respectively). These results suggest the critical incidents in the case contribute distinct information beyond that available from performance ratings.

Three major research studies confirm the reliability and validity of the ABEM certification program (i.e., the written and oral examinations) and support the theory of intelligence that posits three types of intelligence—general, academic, and practical.

Conclusions

The ABEM oral examination is a standardized oral examination using actual clinical scenarios with identified critical incidents. Research findings support the contention that the oral examination assesses several components of practical intelligence, including clinical reasoning. The richness of the unique information gathered in the oral examination and the efficient, reliable, and valid integration of this information into examiners' judgments are notable advantages of this type of performance assessment.

References

1. Sternberg RJ, Wagner RK. The geocentric view of intelligence and job performance is wrong. *Curr Dir in Psychol Sci;* 1993; 2:1-5.

2. Jensen AR. Test validity: *g* versus "tacit knowledge." *Curr Dir in Psychol Sci;* 1993;2:9-10.

3. Ree MJ; Earles JA. *g* is to psychology what carbon is to chemistry: A reply to Sternberg and Wagner, McClelland, and Calfee. *Curr Dir Psychol Sci;* 1993; 2:11-12.

4. Schmidt FL; Hunter JE. Tacit knowledge, practical intelligence, general mental ability, and job knowledge. *Curr Dir Psychol Sci;* 1993; 2; 8-9.

5. Maatsch JL; Munger BS; Podgorny G. On the reliability and validity of the board examination in emergency medicine. In Wolcott BW & Rund DA , (Eds.) *Emergency Medicine Annual 1982.* Norwalk, CN: Appleton-Century-Crofts.

6. Maatsch JL; Huang R; Downing S; Barker D. Predictive Validity of Medical Specialty Examination: Executive Summary. East Lansing, MI: Michigan State University, College of Human Medicine, Office of Medical Education Research and Development. 1993 (monograph)

7. Reinhart MA; Hollenbeck JR; Tuttle DB; Munger BS; Bridgham RG. The Contributions of the Oral Examination Constructs to ABEM Certification. Paper presented at Soc Acad Emerg Med Washington, D.C. (May, 1994).

8. Solomon DJ; Reinhart MA; Bridgham RG; Munger BS Starnamon S. An Assessment of an Oral Examination Format for Evaluating Clinical Competence in Emergency Medicine *Acad Med*; 1990; 65: S43-S44.

Disadvantages to Using the Oral Examination

Robert O. Guerin, Ph.D.
The American Board of Pediatrics

My task this morning is to explore disadvantages of the oral examination. Dr. Mary Ann Reinhart has discussed the advantages of the oral examination and later today others will discuss enhancements and alternatives. Perhaps surprisingly, I happen to agree with Dr. Reinhart about the advantages of the oral examination and can think of other good things about the oral examination. However, well prepared examination procedures may not apply to all evaluation problems. In some cases circumstances or requirements (adequate written examination logistics) may attenuate the value of the oral examination. It is easy to imagine an oral examination that closely simulates the actual practice environment of the physician. The closer this relationship the more likely the oral examination will be useful. Based on recent meetings, the oral examinations of the American Board of Pathology and the American Board of Radiology come to mind. On the other hand, I can also imagine the oral examination as an ineffective substitute for better, more efficient methods of evaluation when the evaluation needs do not match the potential capabilities of the oral examination.

My focus this morning is on a single factor that may explain many potential problems with the oral examination. After defining this factor there will be a review of the experience of the American Board of Pediatrics (ABPeds) with the oral examination. The disadvantages of the oral examination will be highlighted and, finally, some alternatives to the oral examination presented.

The greatest difficulty in oral examination implementation is related to standardization. There are other problems that must be addressed and indeed might amplify the main problem if standardization is deficient, e.g., logistics and cost.

One useful definition of standardization, slightly paraphrased from an article related to multiple choice question (MCQ) testing by Hassmén and Hunt,[1] follows:

> Standardizing means that each examinee is exposed to the *same or equivalent tasks*, which are administered under the *same conditions*, in the *same amount of time*, and with *scoring as objective* as possible.
>
> Three factors control standardization:
>
> 1. Equivalent tasks
> 2. Equivalent conditions
> 3. Objectivity

These factors, if met, underlay all the advantages of an oral examination. Each, if not met, result in disadvantages and discourage the use of the oral. A brief review of the American Board of Pediatrics' experience with the oral examination may add appropriate background for a discussion of both disadvantages and alternatives to the oral examination.

The American Board of Pediatrics' Experience

The American Board of Pediatrics (AB Peds) used an oral examination or similar format since the board's creation in 1933 until 1989. The exam evolved over time to meet the measurement needs of the board and incorporated advances in oral examination design. Oral examination tasks were written and standardized; conditions, both in terms of the examiners and sites, were uniform; and objective data gathering and standard-setting methods were employed.

The first study of the AB Peds' oral examination was commissioned in 1975 and was conducted by the National Board of Medical Examiners (NBME). The study was conducted again in 1976 by the NBME and confirmed the results of the first study. The results indicated that marginally passing examinees on the written examination failed the oral examination at a rate exceeding 67 percent, and that examinees scoring three-fourths of a standard deviation (SD) above the reference group mean passed the oral 100 percent of the time on the first attempt (recent graduates of American medical schools taking the exam for the first time). The results were based on data gathered from nearly 3,000 examinee performance reports.

The NBME recommendations in 1976 were to:

1. Raise the standard for the written examination to 0.3 standard deviations.
2. Excuse from the oral examination those examinees with very high written examination scores.

The board increased the written standard by 0.3 SD in 1976 but did not excuse examinees from the oral.

The next investigation of the oral examination was conducted in 1986 by the American Board of Pediatrics. Nearly 3,400 written and oral examination results were analyzed. The results were similar to those of the earlier studies, and it was recommended and accepted in 1986 that the written standard be increased again by 0.3 SD.

The last oral examination study was conducted in 1988 by the AB Peds. In this study over 21,000 examinee results were analyzed. The study focused upon the overall failure rate of the oral examination over time. In a sense the board was investigating the question, "What did the oral examination do?"

Of the 21,061 examinees' records reviewed between 1976 and 1986, 21.3 percent (4,479) of the examinees were not certified and had no history of taking an oral examination. (See Figure 1.) Of this group, 75 percent had not passed the written examination, while 25 percent had passed the written but had not attempted to take an oral examination.

After accounting for this group of 21.3 percent, 16,582 examinees remained. Of this number, 92.8 percent (15,387) were certified and 7.2 percent (1,175) were not certified.

Of the certified group 92.5 percent passed on the first attempt at the oral examination, 99.4 percent passed after two attempts, 99.9 percent passed after three attempts, and 100 percent passed after four attempts. Only 96 examinees of 15,387 did not pass on the first two attempts. A similar history applies to those not certified in that a vast majority of the non-certified had only taken one oral examination. Past experience suggested that less than one-half of one percent would not be certified after two oral examinations.

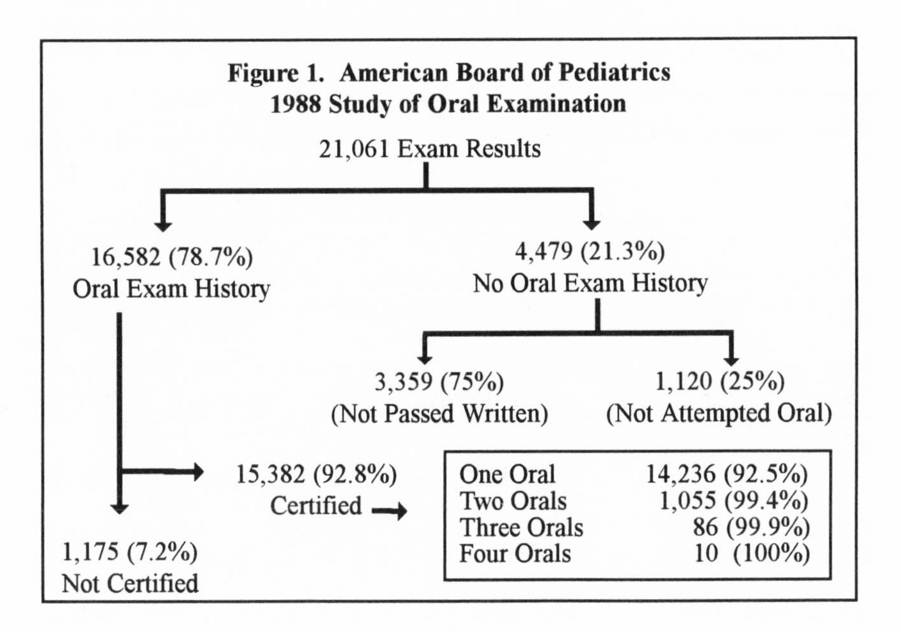

On the basis of these results, a well organized, carefully prepared, and objective oral examination just did not appear to provide the AB Peds with additional information about the examinees. Could it be that the first failure on the oral examination "frightened" the examinees (the "trial by fire" approach) enough to cause them to "study hard." That was one explanation, but it was noted that the written examination did not have that effect. Consistent failure rates for repeat written examinees of 10 percent to 12 percent had been observed over the same time frame as this study. It was generally agreed that the oral examination was well prepared but that after two attempts examinees got the right combination of content and examiners, and they passed.

In addition to being prompted by the results of all three studies, the board considered eliminating the oral because of logistic problems. The number of candidates for general certification had grown significantly, particularly during the time period of the last study. This trend continued through 1994, which was a record year for number of examinees. It became progressively more difficult to arrange and coordinate six oral examination sessions per year for 2,500 examinees. In addition, and certainly the least consideration, the cost of the oral examination was not recovered by the fee; costs were increasing faster than the fee.

Given the study results, logistical problems and cost, the AB Peds dropped the oral examination in 1988. This was accomplished without problems. It should be pointed out that, rather than simply deleting the oral examination, the types of information desired and presumably gathered during the oral examination were defined, the resulting evaluation goals were added to the general certifying process. Also, loss of the frequent meetings by the board with the oral examiners was noted and other arrangements had to be made in order to continue these valuable meetings.

Advantages and Disadvantages

What are disadvantages of the oral examination other than those identified by the American Board of Pediatrics? The disadvantages have the same names as the advantages. In fact, rather than using the term "disadvantage," possibly they should be referred to as "areas of caution." Each area of weakness can be an area of strength. Further, areas of weakness can be recognized and controlled for, to some degree, as will be reported by the next speakers. The disadvantages, or areas of caution, may be categorized into six areas. This categorization is arbitrary, based on my own views of the issue. Others may see more or less, and categorize differently; the more views of the problem the better.

The categories of disadvantages or "areas of caution" are:

1. *Examiner*
2. *Examinee*
3. *Material*
4. *Scoring*
5. *Validity*
6. *Cost and logistics*

Each will be discussed in turn.

Examiner

Examiners provide a great opportunity for the interruption of standardization. Remember the requirements for equivalent tasks, equivalent conditions, and objectivity. For an examiner an oral examination is long, difficult, and at times boring. Moods change and initial impressions and expectations will influence the examiner and, therefore, the examinee. Many variables related to human interaction during an oral examination could be considered. Thus, standardization requires examiners to have:

1. Initial training.
2. Frequent retraining.
3. Limited number of examining sessions.
4. Counseling if systematic bias is detected (examiners who are hawks or doves).
5. Guidance relative to attention and persistence.
6. A clear understanding of the oral examination measurement objectives.

Examinee

The examinee also can play a role in disrupting standardization. This might include:

1. Language problems which can shorten the examination and cause examiner frustration.
2. Prior knowledge of case material or the examiner.
3. Inappropriate understanding of the objectives of the oral examination.
4. Examinee anxiety unrelated to actual competence but related to interacting with an examiner.

Material

Examination material may be the most critical area requiring great caution and effort. The degree of caution depends very much on the structure and timing of the examination. A single examination administration requires less material and may eliminate the need for multiple sets of equivalent material. A single event does not, however, relieve the burden for multiple equivalent material for future examinations. Examination material should:

1. Be equal within a testing period.
2. Be equal across testing periods for a given administration.
3. Be equal across administrations.
4. Be presented in a consistent manner across examiners.
5. Assess material not readily examined using other objective formats.
6. Be relevant.
7. Be varied.

Scoring

Scoring of an oral examination is, because of its nature, a subjective process. Changing conditions, variable case material, examiner comfort, and examiner style all contribute to the subjectivity of the process. Several areas requiring caution include:

1. Explicit rules and criteria for grading.
2. Explicit identification of important measurement data for case material.
3. Decisions about the influence of a single examiner.
4. Explicit rules governing uncertain outcomes both for a single judge and team judgment.
5. Varying examination length due to varying presentations and varying responses.

Validity

Measurement validity is frequently defined as the instrument doing what it was intended to do. It has also been noted that validity can only be confirmed by empirical studies. The word "valid" is defined as something that is well grounded, just, effective, or allows a correct conclusion from a premise.

Validity, for the oral examination, is based on standardization. It provides a well grounded, just, well-known scale which is the most important issue when obtaining data and making a decision. If the scale is unknown or unclear, then the measurements and the subsequent decisions are also unclear. Standardization allows consistent measurement on a known scale which is defined by the oral examination and also sensible generalizations (pass/fail decisions). This is simply the process completed during any examination.

Costs and Logistics

Cost may be the least important factor, but it is a factor that can cause the end of a very good examination. Cost, of course, includes preparation of material, reimbursement of examiners, and the cost of the examination site, as well as scoring, analysis, and reporting. There are also costs for the examinee for travel, hotel, food, and time away from practice. One must be cautious when assessing the value of the examination to ensure that the examination is associated with a fair cost.

Logistics, while appearing routine, are critical; lack of thorough implementation can severely reduce the effectiveness of the examination. The process of getting material to the site and back need not be discussed here, but there are other areas of administration to which attention must be drawn:

1. Adequate time for grading and review.
2. Scheduling time and sessions to allow examinees who know examiners to be shifted to another examiner.
3. Adequate time to train examiners.

American Board of Pediatrics' Alternatives to the Oral Examination

When the American Board of Pediatrics discontinued the oral examination, other areas of the certification process were expanded. It was supposed from the outset that the oral examination had been measuring certain things; thus, for example, part of the oral examination was designed to measure recognition and processing of clinical information. These components are now assessed in an expanded written examination.

In addition to expanding the written examination, the board developed a resident tracking and evaluation system. Residents are evaluated by the residency program director on several points of clinical competence during each of three residency years. In addition to an overall rating regarding the suitability of the candidate to be examined, the program director rates the candidate's data gathering, management and interpersonal skills as well as work habits and personal qualities. Minimum ratings are required before the candidate can take the written examination.

Other Alternatives not Chosen by the American Board of Pediatrics

Other alternatives have been suggested to substitute for or supplement the oral examination. The board has considered but is not using at present:

1. Computer-based simulations
2. OSCE (Objective Structured Clinical Examination)
3. Simulated patients
4. Computer exam supplements during the oral examination
5. Practice evaluation
6. Record review
7. Essay examinations
8. Peer review
9. Patient satisfaction
10. Multiple Hurdle Examination/Sequential Testing

Conclusion

In conclusion, the degree to which an organization fails to standardize an oral examination is the degree to which the advantages of the oral examination become disadvantages. Equivalent tasks, equivalent conditions, and objectivity must be the fundamental components one must consider. Based on the American Board of Pediatrics' experience, even if all else appears satisfactory, a board must consider whether the exam is measuring anything extra, i.e., do the oral examinations obtain information on a scale that improves the understanding of the examinee's capabilities. If that is not the case, a well organized, standardized oral examination may simply be a burden to a board and the examinee without noticeable reward.

References

1. Hassmén P and Hunt DP. Human self-assessment in multiple-choice testing. *J Educ Measure,* 1994 31:149-160.

Discussion

Dr. Elliott L. Mancall (Conference Moderator): The floor is now open. Please identify yourself.

Dr. Fred Jacobs (President, New Jersey State Board of Medical Examiners): I have some questions for the panel on the application of oral examinations because it comes before us quite often. I must tell you that I have a bias against this examination because of the experience we've had. The issues that were raised, particularly by Dr. Reinhart, as to unique information that's obtained about interpersonal factors, emotional control. I ask you how are you able to standardize the kind of assessment you need so as to rank people to draw the line, how much emotional control is required, or how much lack of emotional control would be judged a fail? Also, I think boards in this country that fail individuals, in the environment in which we live now, will be given the opportunity to defend their actions in a court of law. My question is what sort of review does the Board of Emergency Medicine give to those who fail the exam and how can you do it in the absence of a permanent record?

Dr. Mancall: Thank you. Dr. Reinhart.

Dr. Mary Ann Reinhart (American Board of Emergency Medicine): It is a relevant and timely question, because we are right now going through such an appeal. The board does have an established appeal process which it's had for many years. Most protests of an outcome of an examination are typically handled in the first or second step of the appeal process. The appeal starts with the candidate's concern going to the chief examiner, a further appeal goes to the test committee, then the Executive Committee of the board, and finally, if the candidate chooses to go the full length, to an appeal panel which is comprised of three individuals who are either directors or senior directors of the board and who, obviously, have had no involvement with the case at any point before this time. Because of the fact that oral exam cases are based on actual Emergency

Department cases and critical incidents are identified, we do have written records of the candidates' examination. They are not verbatim, and obviously they are not video taped. But, part of the examiners' training is very stringent on monitoring behavior and keeping notes. We do not keep the candidates' notes because they can comprise a variety of different things from scribbling and thinking out loud to what they actually did. But the examiners record on a form every request for information about a case a candidate makes, and their responses, as well as a minute-by-minute timing during the fifteen-minute period. That is one set of notes the board keeps, including outstanding comments, particularly around negative actions that the candidate has made or actions of failure or poor performance. The rating sheet itself has three areas on it: (1) the actual ratings; (2) the examiners' notation about the candidates' performance on the critical incidents which are a key part of this sheet and part of the record, and (3) the examiners' notes on the primary areas of failure or exceptional performance. If the candidate performed some activities in an exceedingly competent manner, those are noted on the form as well. In the last five to eight years the board directors have worked very hard at training examiners and reviewing these notes. As part of the examination, the chief examiners review these notes and all cases and often question the examiners and challenge them to bring them all, hopefully, into conformance.

Dr. Bernard-M. LeFebevre (The Royal College of Physicians and Surgeons of Canada): What I have to say follows very logically on the previous question. We have noticed that over the last four years, since the College introduced a review mechanism into the exam process, that practically all of the requests for review arise from the oral examination. That is the best test that I know for the examination as it stands right now in the College. There have been 55 requests for review; I don't use the word appeals, because I don't want to invite lawyers into the process. It's an extension really of the examination process, and therefore is not judicial, or a quasi-legal process. However, what is questioned by the candidates who request a review is not so much the process itself, but how it is applied by the examiners. Or, how it is applied by the particular specialty that uses the oral examination. Talking about whether the oral is good or bad, or what the advantages or disadvantages of the oral are, is not relevant. The issue really is how is it applied, how is it used? How competent are the examiners in using this particular measurement tool? I would like to have the reaction of the panel about not so much whether the oral is a good or bad examination, but whether the oral exam is used to advantage by the boards who use it?

Dr. Reinhart: I think that the issues that have just been raised are at the heart of the examination process. Standardization of examiners, as well as standardization of the cases and the format, is absolutely critical. The Board of Emergency Medicine's appeal procedure, protest procedure, does allow extensive appeals which have lasted as long as three years. There also is a mechanism for appeal of the content and that was the circumstance that I referred to earlier, we are now going through. It has happened once before in the past seven years; in that circumstance a case was thrown out at the final appeal level. It's difficult to say how far the current process will continue or where it will end. But it is certainly a major issue to be considered and it certainly does absorb the resources of the board, there's no question about it.

Dr. Victor W. Waymouth (College of Physicians & Surgeons of British Columbia, Canada): I ultimately want to ask a question of both Dr. Reinhart and Dr. Page, but perhaps a little bit of a preamble. We have a term in Canada to describe a certain kind of physician, what we often say is that "he knows the words, but he doesn't know the music." What I'm hearing is a considerable amount of attention played to the words and not necessarily getting us to whether the physician can actually sing the song. It's a little bit of a distinction between competence and performance. I think what I heard Dr. Page say, although he didn't actually use the word "performance," but stressed focusing on the clinical decision, was the ultimate translation of all that went before, and to see whether in fact they can, in the end, perform. I'd like to ask if that is a correct interpretation. Is the concept of trying to get at the clinical decision an attempt to move closer to what the actual performance is like in the real setting?

I would also like to ask Dr. Reinhart, you refer to the fact, if I understood it correctly, that the best predictor of *performance* was measurement of the three types of intelligence. Along the same theme, I would suggest that the best predictor of *competence* is the three types of intelligence, but you left out the critical factor of the motivation of the physician to, in fact, apply the competence. We in Canada are trying to get closer and closer to the performance and moving, in a sense, away from the components leading to competence. Dr. Page, is your comment that we should move closer to performance rather than the components of competence? Dr. Reinhart, did I understand you correctly?

Dr. Mancall: Thank you. In view of the musical quality of that question, I don't know if you two want to orchestrate the response. Dr. Page, do you want to respond initially?

Dr. Gordon G. Page (The University of British Columbia): I think it would be our desire always to assess performance, but I do not think we are doing that. Any time people are placed in a contrived situation, whether it be a written examination or an oral examination, we are measuring their ability to do something which is their competence. I guess a clinical decision is one step closer to what they might do in a real situation, but it is still a contrived situation, so I don't think we are measuring performance.

Dr. Reinhart: I very much appreciate your comment about motivation, you did understand correctly what I said. It is an issue for the board and the board has considered it but not to the level of implementation as yet. It has considered how it might look at other components of actual performance of an emergency physician. Clearly one of them is motivation. Everyone is motivated in a testing situation when certification is the outcome, particularly with the changes in the last five years about the importance of certification. I do not think the board could claim to be measuring motivation. Perhaps a better way to do that might be to follow the lead of the Board of Pediatrics and work with the residency programs to obtain some measure during the residency.

Dr. Frank L. Thorne (American Board of Plastic Surgery): I wanted to differentiate a little bit between standardization and fairness, both absolutely required in the examinations of each individual candidate. But I wanted to caution against trying to extrapolate standardization too much across boards. If you think about it, each board, in effect, turns out different products. The requirements of one board for competency are not necessarily those of another. For instance, in my fairly small specialty, in addition to needing cognitive knowledge the board must also evaluate mechanical skills, and, even if I dare say so, cosmetic judgment. These are skills that in our board's estimation cannot ever be judged purely on a written examination; that's why the discourse with an experienced oral examiner is essential, using his/her own judgement to be sure, hopefully, in a semi-standardized way to evaluate a candidate. What may be good for our board and necessary for our board may not be true in all specialties.

Dr. Robert O. Guerin (American Board of Pediatrics): That is a great point. I did not want to be misinterpreted as stating that one should standardize everything out of existence in oral exams. I think there will be a variety, variance, within the process of standardizing, so that each examinee receives the same types of approach, and the same types of data are gathered. Certainly there will be variability across boards, across examinees, and across examiners. Sometimes one has to know that and control for it, sometimes take advantage of it, and sometimes one cannot do a thing about it because it is the special interest of the discipline.

Dr. Gerald P. Whelan (American Board of Emergency Medicine): I am very familiar with the ABEM examination that Dr. Reinhart so eloquently described. Our board truly believes that the oral exam does test something that is different from the written examination in terms of critical decisions, what we call critical actions. In fact, often in working with examiners we de-emphasize the need to explore the candidates' thinking and rationale for the decision, and focus on whether the decision is appropriately made. My question is basically that Dr. Guerin's presentation did not make it clear to me the nature of the pediatric board's oral examination; whether it tested critical decisions, or whether it was an oral exam retesting of what Dr. Reinhart called "academic knowledge." It is obviously possible to fashion an oral examination which essentially takes a written examination and makes it oral, with basically the same material, the same emphasis. My first question is for Dr. Guerin: Could you briefly describe the nature of the pediatric oral examination? Then a general question for the panel: are we really talking about a single entity here when speaking about the oral examination, or are there substantial differences between different board exams? Comparing oral and written examinations may have varying validity depending on the design of both tests.

Dr. Guerin: The American Board of Pediatrics' oral exam for the ten or fifteen years before it was discontinued consisted of four 30-minute sessions with one examiner each. The examiners acted as a team to develop final grading after the two hours was complete. It included one 30-minute session which we called the graphics laboratory section, an array of 15 or 20 selections of graphic material or laboratory information with a developed, edited, standardized protocol related to the questions and responses that should come from the examinee. The second session was a series of mini-cases; a brief medical history with the intent of assigning a diagnosis or steps in management. And finally, two half-hour sessions that were very open-ended, just a simple opening vignette related to a patient, with three, four or five vignettes within each session. Each examiner was required to get through at least three vignettes. It seemed to sample an array of topics in pediatrics. I think that over time the board just kept feeling it was measuring the candidate's memory of the words and not ever sure about the music.

Dr. Page: My general comment is that perhaps more than anything else a board does, the examination they deliver conveys the board's value system to candidates. Within orals there are opportunities to assess things that cannot be assessed with written examinations, procedural skills, interpersonal skills, clinical skills and so on. I think that is a direct message to your candidates about what is important.

Dr. Mark L. Dyken (American Board of Psychiatry & Neurology): I suppose I wanted to say exactly what you're saying and, at the risk of being repetitious, saying the same thing I did last year at the conference. At Indiana University when we were trying to compare variabilities in correlation of course performance, I took a look at what medical students did in chemistry and anatomy. There's a very close correlation between performance in these courses. If you follow some of the reasoning given today, you might decide if they do well on chemistry, to drop anatomy.

Dr. Edward R. Ames (American Veterinary Medical Association): I have a question for Dr. Reinhart: How many candidates are examined each year and how many examiners are involved in the process?

Dr. Reinhart: We have about 570 candidates at one examination, which is held over the course of three days. There are two half-day sessions each day, for a total of six sessions. We have about 125 examiners who are present to conduct the exam.

Dr. Ames: And how many diplomates are in your specialty?

Dr. Reinhart: I believe it's about 13,000.

Dr. Page: Just a question really which is more difficult to defend, a system that is less reliable, very subjective and so on, as we seem to think oral exams are (and I think that is correct), or to defend a system based on a written examination which is highly reliable, but for which, I think, we don't have any really good evidence of a direct link between performance on a written examination and performance as a specialist?

PART 4

RECENT ADVANCES IN THE STANDARDIZED ORAL EXAMINATION

Standardization of the Examination Process

Balancing Validity and Reliability by Using Live Patients

The Construct Validity of an Oral Examination

Recent Changes in the Obstetrics and Gynecology Oral Examination

Assumptions in Scoring Oral Examinations

Statistical Methods to Improve Decision Reproducibility

Discussion

Standardization of the Examination Process

Francis P. Hughes, Ph.D.
The American Board of Anesthesiology

Background

The American Board of Anesthesiology (ABA) issues its certificate to those who demonstrate that they meet its standard for certification as a consultant in anesthesiology. The board defines the qualities of a consultant anesthesiologist as:

> A physician who possesses knowledge, judgment, adaptability, clinical skills, technical facility and personal characteristics sufficient to carry out the entire scope of anesthesiology practice. A consultant is able to communicate effectively with peers, patients, their families and others involved in the medical community. The consultant anesthesiologist can serve as an expert in matters related to anesthesiology, deliberate with others and provide advice and defend opinions in all aspects of the specialty. An ABA diplomate is able to function as the leader of the anesthesiology care team.[1]

The consultant anesthesiologist must be able to manage emergent life-threatening situations in an independent and timely fashion. The ability to acquire and process information in an independent and timely manner is central to assure individual responsibility for all aspects of anesthesiology care. Adequate physical and sensory faculties and coordinated function of the extremities are essential, as are freedom from the influence of or dependency on chemical substances that impair cognition, physical, sensory, or motor functions.

The ABA certification process is designed to assess whether candidates possess these qualities. Today, and for some time in the past, training programs attest to the board that the graduating resident is able to practice anesthesiology safely and independently. The credentialing and examination components of the ABA process ensure that candidates for certification possess the qualities of a consultant anesthesiologist.

The examination component was comprised of a written, an oral, and a practical examination when the board was formed initially in 1937. In the practical examination the examiners were expected to "observe the work of candidates in their own or similar operating room surroundings, their relations to other staff members, and investigate their professional standing."[2] It was a practical demonstration of the candidate's clinical practice which might include ". . . inspection of clinical records, records of departmental activities, library facilities, available apparatus; and demonstrations of application of anesthetic agents, methods and techniques included in Anesthesiology."[3]

By the 1950s the ABA introduced a survey examination and, at its discretion, required some but not all candidates to give a practical demonstration of their anesthesiology practice. The ABA discontinued the practical examination by 1960 and the survey examination in 1977. Although the examination component had changed significantly, the certification process continued to retain many of the elements of the original, but in a different and more standardized form.

In the mid-1950s the ABA began to require that candidates submit annual reports of their anesthesia experiences to the board. These reports eventually led to the requirement in 1977 that all training programs file a semiannual Clinical Competence Committee (CCC) Report for every resident, using evaluation guidelines and a form provided by the ABA. The CCC report is an evaluation of those elements of a resident's performance and professional and ethical standing previously assessed by the practical or survey examination.

The oral examination evolved to its present form during this period of change as well. Initially, it covered the same subjects as the written examination but emphasized their clinical application. It continues to emphasize the application of scientific principles to clinical practice in all phases of anesthesiology, but has been designed to assess many of the qualities originally assessed by the practical examination.

Standardization of the certification process has been paramount almost from the beginning. Initially, efforts were directed to assure, as noted above, that the ABA assessed every candidate's knowledge and clinical skill at the level of a practicing anesthesiologist. Three assessment components in the certification process are used currently:

1. **The Clinical Competence Committee Report**. An assessment at the completion of the anesthesia residency to establish that the candidate has the essential attributes, knowledge, acquired character skills (e.g., adaptable and flexible, careful and thorough, appropriately self-confident), judgment, and clinical skills necessary to practice anesthesiology safely and independently.

2. **The written examination**. The test is designed to measure the candidate's knowledge base and cognitive and deductive skills.
3. **The oral examination**. The oral is designed to evaluate the candidate's ability to manage patients as presented in clinical scenarios.

The CCC reports are in large measure a standardized assessment conducted by the residency program faculty of the resident's ability to practice anesthesiology, and the written examination provides a standard measure of knowledge of the discipline for all candidates. I wish today to describe the efforts to standardize the ABA oral examination process.

Oral Examination Objectives

The ABA designed and developed its oral examination to assess the candidate's decision-making skills, with particular emphasis on the scientific and clinical rationale that led to the decisions. It uses the examination to evaluate a candidate's ability to manage surgical and anesthetic complications, and other unexpected clinical changes. The candidate is expected to recognize the pertinent aspects of the clinical scenario, make rational diagnoses and develop appropriate treatment protocols. The oral examination also affords the candidate the opportunity to demonstrate the ability to communicate effectively.

Examination Content

The core of the ABA oral examination is the "guided question," with supplemental "additional topics." Each examination session is based on one guided question and three additional topics. The same guided question and additional topics are used simultaneously in all examining rooms. A different guided question and additional topics are used for each half-hour session. The examination content is thus identical for all candidates being examined at the same time.

The guided question consists of a stem and a series of major subsections for consideration in conducting the examination. The stem is an abbreviated case description of a problem in anesthetic management. The subsections comprise preoperative evaluation, intraoperative course, and postoperative care.

The additional topics are unrelated to the guided question, being inserted to provide breadth to the examination. The ABA carefully matches the two guided questions and six additional topics that comprise a candidate's examination in order to minimize overlap in content and to assure that the total examination has appropriate depth and adequate scope of content.

Examination Format

All candidates have two consecutive 30-minute examination sessions. Approximately ten minutes before each session candidates receive a written statement of the stem for the guided question to help them organize their thoughts about the case. A different pair of examiners conducts each session. The senior and junior examiner in each pair are assigned specific areas of the examination.

The senior examiner has five minutes at the beginning of the examination session to question the candidate about the preoperative preparations for the case. The junior examiner then questions the candidate for the next 15 minutes about the intraoperative phase and postoperative care of the patient. Finally, the senior examiner uses at least two of the additional topics during the last ten minutes to add breadth to the examination. If the senior examiner deems it appropriate, this time is also used to explore in more depth aspects of the intraoperative and postoperative elements of the guided question.

At the end of each session the two examiners independently assign the candidate a grade. ABA staff then collects the examiners' grade reports. Upon completion of two half-hour sessions there are four independent assessments of each candidate.

Early in the evolution of the oral examination the ABA examiners used material from their own practice experience as the basis for questioning the candidates, selecting their own topics to give breadth to the examination. There was anecdotal evidence to justify the euphemistic comment that some of these topics were "zingers." The ABA then defined for the senior examiners a set of suggested topics to use at their discretion after the case discussion to augment the scope of the examination; in time the optional suggested topics became mandatory additional topics which the ABA matches to the guided questions to provide balance as well as breadth.

The ABA believes that the technique of using guided questions and additional topics provides uniformity of oral examination content throughout each examination. The oral examination tests the candidate's ability to organize and utilize information, make judgments, adapt to changing and unexpected events, and communicate her or his line of reasoning and basis for decisions.

Examiner Selection and Training

The ABA receives nominations for associate examiners from a number of sources. It solicits recommendations about the nominees from diplomates who not only know the nominee but also are board examiners. The purpose of the vetting process is to ascertain whether the nominees possess the personal qualities that are necessary to serve as an associate examiner.

Every associate examiner receives the *Handbook for Associate Examiners of the American Board of Anesthesiology.* In addition to providing background information about the ABA, including ABA policies pertaining to associate examiners, the handbook includes an overview of the board's certification process and a description of candidate deficiencies and responses. The handbook includes a description of the examination standard and the attributes of a consultant anesthesiologist.

All new examiners are required to participate in a 2.5-hour workshop conducted by several ABA directors the day before they begin examining candidates. The ABA may require other examiners to attend the workshop if they have not conducted oral examinations for the board in the last two years. Other, relatively inexperienced examiners may choose to attend the workshop on a voluntary basis.

The workshop for new examiners begins with an overview of the ABA certification process, a discussion about the attributes of a consultant anesthesiologist and guidance as to how to recognize each attribute during the oral examination. Directors discuss the appropriate use of the "guided question" and explain the grading process. They demonstrate appropriate techniques for examining candidates who may have different response styles; directors and new examiners role-play candidate and examiner, respectively, so the new examiners can recognize the issues discussed in the workshop and practice appropriate examination techniques.

An ABA director is assigned as a preceptor to one new examiner, observing and counseling the new examiner throughout the examination week. The preceptor and other directors evaluate a new examiner's potential to develop as an associate examiner and provide reports to the board. Twenty percent of new examiners do not achieve associate examiner status.

A refresher workshop is also conducted for experienced examiners before each week of oral examinations.

Examiner Grading

Each examiner rates the candidate's performance on all aspects of the oral examination. For each area of questioning the examiners record their ratings about the candidate's judgment, adaptability, application of scientific and clinical principles, and ability to communicate effectively. The ABA does not assign specific weights to the different areas of the examination. Examiners are instructed to weigh the candidate's performance against the qualities of a consultant anesthesiologist and assign one of four grades (70, 73, 77 and 80).

A grade of 80 means the examiner is confident that the candidate has demonstrated the qualities of a consultant anesthesiologist during the examination, while a grade of 70 means the candidate clearly did not demonstrate these qualities. The grades of 73 and 77 are used when the examiner is uncertain about the candidate's consultant qualities because the examination did not elicit sufficient information. The examiners are instructed to use one of the extreme grades if there is no doubt about the candidate's qualities. The four-point grading scale is not a high/low, pass/fail system.

A candidate's examination score is the average of the four examiners' grades. The same weight is given to the senior and junior examiners' grades when computing the average. Scores are not adjusted on the basis of other information about the candidate. An average score of 75.1 or greater is required to pass the oral examination. At least two examiners must give the candidate a failing grade for the candidate to fail the examination.

Monitoring and Counseling Examiners

Current and former ABA directors monitor the performance of associate examiners. When not examining candidates, directors audit senior examiners in terms of both examination technique and grading. The Chair of the Examinations Committee reviews the audit reports as they are received throughout the examination week, using the information to counsel the examiner subsequently through correspondence. Informal counseling sessions may be held during the examination week. A summary report is kept of the audits for each examiner, with a cumulative summary being used by the board when deciding to retain or promote examiners.

The ABA also analyzes examination data to obtain information about the frequency of outlier events for each examiner. An outlier event occurs when the grades a candidate receives from the examiners in one room differ by seven or ten (i.e., 70 and 77) and the grades the candidate receives from the examiners in the other room differ by at most, three (i.e., 80 and 77). In this example, the examiner who gave a grade of 70 is an outlier. Examiners who frequently are outliers either do not have a clear understanding of the standard for certification or they have an understanding that is at variance with that of the directors and their fellow examiners.

Candidate Orientation

The ABA urges all residency programs to conduct practice oral examinations for their residents and recent graduates to ensure that all candidates have an equal opportunity to prepare for the oral examination. To assist programs to provide practice examinations in the board format, the ABA invites a small number of residency program directors to a workshop for non-examiners.

Prior to the examination, the ABA sends candidates the following to inform them about the oral examination process:

1. A description of the oral examination process.
2. A sample guided question and additional topics.
3. A description of the attributes of a consultant anesthesiologist and a list of common deficiencies.

In an attempt to alleviate the candidates' examination anxiety, examination facilities are selected in urban and resort settings that will afford the candidates comfortable accommodations with a minimum of distractions. Former ABA directors register the candidates at the examination site. As pointed out previously, candidates receive the stem for each guided question approximately ten minutes before the individual session begins. There is a chair and writing board outside each examination room for candidates to sit and organize their thoughts. The intent of these efforts is to reduce extraneous factors that might have an adverse impact on examination performance. Candidates are assigned to examiners who do not know them and have not examined them previously.

Summary

The ABA seeks to ensure that the oral examination fulfills its assessment objectives and provides a fair examination to all candidates. Efforts are made to standardize the examination by controlling the format and content, informing candidates about the process prior to the oral examination, selecting and monitoring the associate examiners, and continually assessing the entire process, including grading procedures. The board is confident that the standardized oral examination in its current form is meeting its objectives.

References

1. *American Board of Anesthesiology, Booklet of Information,* 1995.
2. *American Board of Anesthesiology, Booklet of Information,* 1937.
3. *American Board of Anesthesiology, Booklet of Information,* 1950.

Balancing Validity and Reliability by Using Live Patients

Stephen C. Scheiber, M.D.
The American Board of Psychiatry and Neurology

The American Board of Psychiatry and Neurology (ABPN) is the only one of the 24 American Board of Medical Specialties (ABMS) Member Boards that uses live patients for examination purposes. As an initial step, candidates must pass a one-day written examination before they can sit for the oral examination. The oral examination in psychiatry is two hours long with a one-hour live patient section. The neurology examination is three hours long, again with one hour devoted to a live patient. Adult neurologists examine an adult patient; child neurologists examine a child. The second hour in psychiatry begins with a videotape of a psychiatrist interviewing a patient, followed by questions regarding the taped case. The other two hours in neurology consist of child and adult vignette sections, with five clinical vignettes per section. To pass the oral examinations, candidates in psychiatry must pass both sections in a single examination. Candidates in neurology must pass all three sections, although not necessarily in one sitting.

The ABPN is often queried as to why live patients remain a part of its oral examinations. The overriding issue has to do with face validity. There are strong feelings in the field that this is the best method to ensure that board certified psychiatrists and neurologists can examine bona fide psychiatric and neurologic patients, discuss their findings, and formulate diagnoses and treatment and management plans in a logical and clinically relevant manner. This examination process has been reviewed on several occasions by the board; each time the board has voted to continue using this assessment method.

To enhance standardization as well as quality control, the board assigns one senior and two primary examiners for each examination hour. The two primary examiners remain in the room at all times with the candidate, while the senior examiner divides his/her time between two rooms during the course of an examination. The primary examiners reach a consensus grade within 20 minutes of completion of the examination with guidance and advice from the senior examiner as required. At the beginning of each hour candidates are told that if they know an examiner they should declare a conflict; another examiner is immediately assigned under such circumstances.

The Examination in Psychiatry

In reviewing a psychiatrist candidate's performance with a psychiatric patient, examiners evaluate the physician-patient relationship, the conduct of the interview, and the organization and presentation of the data. Since the patient-doctor relationship is such an integral part of the practice of psychiatry, examiners focus on the candidate's ability to establish rapport and to be empathic and responsive to the patient during the course of the interview.

In conducting the examination, examiners are interested in how candidates elicit information, how they follow up on leads from the patient, the thoroughness of the questioning, and the comprehensiveness of the examination which should include not only symptomatic behaviors and signs of an illness but also the psychological and social aspects of a patient's history. The patient interview must progress in an orderly, logical fashion.

There are many reasons for failing the clinical oral examination in psychiatry as enumerated in Figure 1.

Figure 1. Commonly cited reasons for failing the clinical (live patient) examination for psychiatry board certification

1. History and mental status examination poorly organized
2. Dismissing patient in less than 30 minutes
3. No time allotted for mental status examination
4. Not establishing rapport with patient
5. Not following up on leads with patient
6. Diffuse, unfocused differential diagnosis
7. Reciting a "laundry list" of diagnoses
8. Lack of coherence in diagnostic investigations
9. Shotgun approach to diagnostic investigations with little prioritization
10. Unfamiliarity with toxicity or with preferred dosages of psychopharmacologic agents

In the live patient encounter, the history and mental status assessments may be poorly organized. A candidate may dismiss a patient in less than the 30 minutes provided and yet not have completed a full examination. A candidate may not allot enough time to do an adequate mental status examination. Some are not able to establish rapport with the assigned patients, or may not be astute at following up on critical leads provided by the patients. Some candidates formulate a diffuse, unfocused differential diagnosis, simply reciting a laundry list of all inclusive diagnoses. Others lack coherence and direction in their diagnostic investigations, employing a "shotgun" approach with little prioritization. Finally, some seem unfamiliar with the toxicity of psychopharmacologic agents or with the preferred dosages of such agents.

The second psychiatric section consists of a 25-minute videotape of a psychiatrist interviewing a psychiatric patient. Candidates are asked what additional information they want to obtain and how the additional information can be used. They must summarize and formulate the case based on the available information and must offer a differential diagnosis and management plan, along with a prognosis. Candidates are graded on the basis of their assessment of phenomenology, diagnosis and prognosis, as well as their discussion regarding etiological, pathogenic and therapeutic issues measured along the axes of biological, psychological and social components.

Reasons for candidate failures in the audiovisual section are much the same as cited in the live patient session and are listed in Figure 2.

Figure 2: Commonly cited reasons for failing the audiovisual examination section for psychiatry board certification

1. Disorganized presentation and formulation
2. Inappropriate differential diagnosis
3. Inability to settle on a single working diagnosis
4. Inability to justify how additional data may be helpful
5. Inability to apply book knowledge to the clinical situation
6. Failure to volunteer enough information to determine that a candidate deserves a passing grade

Candidates are often disorganized in their presentation and formulation of the case. They may provide an incomplete list of differential diagnoses or be unable to settle on a single working diagnosis. They may be unable to justify how additional data may be helpful and sometimes cannot apply book knowledge to the particular clinical situation. They may fail to present enough information about the case to pass.

In a study reported by McDermott[1] the rate of agreement on the initial grades assigned by the two primary examiners ranged from 64 percent to 67 percent during a one-year cycle of three examinations involving 2,842 examinations. Weighted Kappas were calculated and ranged from 0.54 to 0.56 representing fair to good agreement beyond chance.

The Examination in Neurology

One hour of the examination in neurology is devoted to a live patient. In general, patients are selected who are capable of providing a history (i.e., cannot be in a coma or severely aphasic) and who preferably exhibit localizing neurologic signs. The candidate is observed while he or she obtains a history and performs the examination. The thoroughness, completeness and precision of the examination of the patient is assessed by the examiners. Neurologists believe strongly that the use of a monitored patient interaction sends a strong message to the training programs about the need for neurology residents to become adept at performing an appropriate neurologic examination. Fortunately, most board candidates have mastered this skill.

Reasons for failing the neurologic patient examination are outlined in Figure 3.

Figure 3. Commonly cited reasons for failing the patient examination for neurology board certification

1. Poor organization of history and physical
2. Insufficient time devoted to history taking
3. Lack of logical progression in physical examination
4. Poor rapport with patient
5. Differential diagnosis with little relevance to case; overly inclusive "laundry list" of diagnoses
6. Diagnostic investigations presented in "shotgun" approach rather than targeting problem presented
7. Failure to know toxicity of neuropharmacologic agents

They include, for example, poor organization of the history and examination with insufficient time devoted to history taking and lack of a logical progression in the physical examination. The examination may be incoherent or fail to elicit significant abnormalities. Poor rapport with the patient or inappropriate behavior can result in candidate failure. Failure also occurs if the differential diagnosis shows little relevance to the case but is overly inclusive without appropriate prioritization. Diagnostic investigations may similarly be suggested in a shotgun manner, that does not target the patient's primary problem. At times, the candidate may possess too little information about the indications for common diagnostic evaluations. Finally, the candidate may be unfamiliar with the toxicity of commonly used neuropharmacologic agents.

The written vignettes that are used in the other two hours of the neurology examination describe a patient with a specific neurologic condition. The candidates may ask the examiner for additional information but must justify the need for the data. As with the live patients, candidates are asked to describe the differential diagnosis, treatment and management for the patient. The last ten minutes of this hour are devoted to issues of critical care in neurology, with exemplary cases provided by the examiners.

As detailed in Figure 4, failure in the vignette sections on the neurology examination reflects a variety of factors, including incomplete knowledge of the particular neurologic disorder; disorganized differential diagnoses; inadequate proposed laboratory or radiologic evaluation for the condition presented; and premature closure in deciding upon the nature of the neurologic problem with an insufficient database. Some candidates cannot apply book knowledge to clinical situations, or there is insufficient information elicited by the candidate or a lack of clarity in arriving at conclusions to justify a passing grade.

Figure 4. Commonly cited reasons for failing the vignette sections of the examination for neurology board certification.

1. Incomplete knowledge of particular neurologic disorders
2. Disorganized differential diagnosis
3. Inadequate laboratory or radiologic evaluation for conditions presented
4. Premature conclusions regarding neurologic problems without sufficient database
5. Failure to apply book knowledge to clinical situation presented
6. Insufficient information presented or lack of clarity to justify a passing grade

The Relationship Between Part I Written and Part II Oral Examination Results

A primary consideration for certifying boards is whether a costly oral examination, which is less reliable than a multiple-choice examination, can be eliminated and either replaced by another method or incorporated into the written examination. One way to assess the significance of such a change would be to compare the results of the written examination with those of the oral examination.

The ABPN has followed a cohort of neurology candidates who took their first Part I examination in April 1990. Of these, 382 (86%) passed Part I after one or more attempts and have taken the Part II exam. The remainder have not repeated Part I, have failed Part I on reexamination, or have passed Part I and not yet attempted Part II.

The cross-tabulation of their first time performance on Part I and on Part II appears in Figure 5.

Figure 5. First attempt on Part I vs. first attempt on Part II for a neurology cohort

	Part I		
Part II	**Pass**	**Fail**	**Total**
Pass	245 (82%)	55 (67%)	300 (79%)
Fail	55 (18%)	27 (33%)	82 (21%)
Total	300 (79%)	82 (21%)	382

Of the 382 who have taken both examinations, 300 (79%) passed Part I on the first attempt and 82 (21%) failed. On Part II, 300 (79%) also passed on the first attempt and 82 (21%) failed. Of the 300 who passed Part I on first attempt, 245 (82%) also passed Part II on first attempt, and 55 (18%) failed. Of the 82 who failed Part I on first attempt, 55 (67%) passed Part II on first attempt and 27 (33%) failed. Chi-square analysis indicated that those candidates who passed Part I on the first attempt also fared better on their first attempt at Part II ($X^2 = 8.14$; d.f. = 1; $p = .004$).

Of particular interest are the 55 candidates who passed Part I on the first attempt but failed Part II on the first attempt. This group scored well above the passing level of 66% for the major examination section (mean = 73%; S.D. = 4.7%) and 60% for the minor section (mean = 74%; S.D. = 5.1%).

These results suggest that raising the Part I standards modestly would not screen out candidates who are likely to fail Part II. A similar study is planned for psychiatry.

The results of the Part II examination have raised challenging questions. In psychiatry the fail rate is higher on the patient section than on the audiovisual section. It is a reasonable guess that the patient section is more highly valued by examiners. In addition, the examiners view 60 minutes of a candidate's performance in the patient section, rather than the 30 minutes of interviews of the audiovisual section after the first 25 minutes are spent by the candidate passively viewing someone else's work. The amount of actual exposure to the candidate may, therefore, be a contributing factor. Yet another concern is, of course, why do candidates fail either the overall psychiatry or neurology examination? A number of reasons have already been cited (Figures 1-4). One discouraging, although not documented, possibility is that, in light of the relative shortage of residency candidates in both psychiatry and neurology, inadequate candidates are recruited into programs to fill empty slots and hence do not represent the best in a large pool of physicians. Another is that programs of marginal quality may be producing marginal psychiatrists and neurologists. Lastly, and also not documented, it is possible that some candidates are so anxious that they cannot conduct an appropriate examination of a patient under our examination conditions, and so are doomed to failure.

In spite of its limitations, the ABPN remains committed to the oral examination, including the use of live patients. We believe that this exercise tests skills, knowledge and a way of thinking critically about clinical issues that is significantly different from what can be tested with a written examination and that a written examination would never be as good for this purpose. Hence, the ABPN is willing to accept the criticism that an oral examination is not perhaps as reliable an examination process as a written examination but believes that the face validity justifies its continuation.

Reference

1. McDermott JF Jr, Tanguay PE, Scheiber SC, et al. Reliability of the Part I board certification examination in psychiatry: Interexaminer consistency. *Am J Psychiatry,* 1991; 148:1672-1674.

The Construct Validity of an Oral Examination

Robert W. Cantrell, M.D.
University of Virginia Medical Center
Byron J. Bailey, M.D.
University of Texas Medical Branch, Galveston

Introduction

Construction and administration of a valid certification examination has always been a goal of the American Board of Otolaryngology (ABOto), a goal subsequently adopted by the American Board of Medical Specialties (ABMS) as well. There is no uniformity among the ABMS Member Boards in this respect, but the process usually consists of a written examination, an oral examination, or a combination of the two. The American Board of Internal Medicine and the American Board of Pediatrics use only a written examination; the surgical boards nearly all use a combination of written and oral examinations. Some boards also use case reviews, and one board still uses actual patients.

The purpose of this communication is to discuss the evolution of the certification process of the American Board of Otolaryngology and to share our recent experience in the use of the oral examination.

History

The concept of standardizing postgraduate medical education and administering an examination to measure the knowledge acquired during that educational process arose within the specialty of otolaryngology. In 1913, at a meeting of the American Laryngological, Rhinological and Otological Society (a.k.a.

the Triological Society), concern was expressed that the various postgraduate educational programs had no uniformity or standardization. In fact, at that time there were no standards, and there was no way for the public to ascertain who had received postgraduate education or to determine the quality of that training. There were some relatively good postgraduate training programs in the U.S. and Europe, but these were mainly preceptorships of unspecified length and variable quality. There were no examinations or other methods of certifying to the public who had or had not completed this additional training.

The concerns of the Triological Society were conveyed to the American Academy of Ophthalmology and Otolaryngology (AAOO) whose leadership appointed two committees, one for ophthalmology and one for otolaryngology, to study the matter. The committee for ophthalmology consisted of representatives from three organizations, the AAOO, the American Ophthalmological Society, and the Ophthalmology Section Council of the American Medical Association (AMA).

They adopted as a goal the creation of a board to administer an examination and award a certificate.

The otolaryngology committee consisted of representatives from five organizations: The American Otological Society, the American Laryngological Association, the Triological Society, the Section Council on Otorhinolaryngology of the AMA and the American Academy of Ophthalmology and Otolaryngology. This group concentrated on standardizing and accrediting postgraduate educational programs and devoted less attention to the examination process as such. This ambitious undertaking may have accounted for the fact that ophthalmology, with only three organizations and a more modest agenda, was able to establish their board and a certification process by 1917, while otolaryngology, on the other hand, dealing with five organizations, standardization and accreditation of programs plus a certification examination, and the delay occasioned by World War I, was not able to establish a board until 1924.

One must appreciate the attitude of physicians at that time. Having had no standardization or controls many, if not most, training programs and physicians were reluctant to submit to a voluntary process developed by "self-appointed" guardians of the public weal. It was into this environment that courageous and farsighted physicians set forth on a quest which by any reasonable measure has succeeded far beyond their expectations. This voluntary process has become so successful that many institutions, particularly hospitals, managed care organizations, and the legal community, impute to it a quality not claimed by the boards themselves. This reputation, plus the many imitators of the process, now threaten its very existence.

The ABOto, incorporated in 1924, maintained its standardization and accreditation mission until 1955 when it turned this task over to the Residency Review Committee for Otolaryngology. This group and its counterparts in other specialties functioned independently until 1971 when the Liaison Committee for Graduate Medical Education (LCGME), later to become the Accreditation Council for Graduate Medical Education (ACGME) was formed.

The establishment of the American Board of Ophthalmology in 1917 and the American Board of Otolaryngology in 1924 was quickly followed by establishment of the American Board of Obstetrics and Gynecology (1930) and the American Board of Dermatology (1932). These four boards joined forces in 1933 in a confederation known as the Advisory Board of Medical Specialties, later to become the American Board of Medical Specialties (ABMS).

Formed initially to share information on how better to evaluate candidates for certification, a function still primary to the organization, the ABMS has grown into a 24 board organization which is preeminent in the world as a voluntary, standard-setting organization dedicated to providing to those needing medical care proof that the physicians they are consulting have completed rigorous, accredited training of a specified length and have successfully passed a carefully constructed examination designed to measure the information gained during their education and training.

The ABMS Member Boards have never claimed to certify competence, and in fact are careful to avoid using that term in connection with the process. Additionally, they have never claimed that someone who has successfully completed this process is more capable than someone who has not. The legal community, however, holds board certified practitioners to a higher standard of practice, and many hospitals and managed care organizations, through their credentialing process, require board certification in order to receive privileges to practice. These requirements, imposed on a voluntary process and never intended by the boards' founders, have focused public, governmental, and legal scrutiny on the process. The voluntary policing of the examination process by the boards themselves over the years has now assumed a dominant position, mandating a careful and frequent evaluation of the process.

The initial certification process utilized by the ABOto consisted of case reviews, a written examination and an oral examination. Subsequently, only the oral examination and live patients were used; in the middle 1970s the board ceased using live patients and began to utilize both written and oral examinations, combining the scores to reach a final score.

As the certifying examinations of the American Board of Otolaryngology were continuously improved, the examination process became increasingly sophisticated and expensive. An examination of higher quality introduced additional costs and placed a significant strain on the finances of the ABOto. It became obvious that there would be a major cost saving if the number of both examiners and candidates for the oral examination could be reduced. This, among other factors, led to the decision to separate the oral and written examinations by several months and to screen out candidates who either scored poorly or extremely well on the written examination. Clearly, this represented a significant change from the pass/fail decision that was based on a *combination* of the written and oral examination scores. It necessitated the selection of points on a continuum of scores that were identified as the low fence (candidates scoring above this level were invited to sit for the oral examination) and the high fence (candidates scoring above this level were certified on the basis of the written examination alone and excused from the oral examination).

This process was cost effective since there were fewer candidates and, hence, fewer examiners required. It soon became apparent, however, that this process led to the perception that there were two classes of diplomates. Some practitioners were stating on their C.V., inappropriately, that they were certified without being required to take an oral examination, as though this somehow placed them in a superior category. Worse, some attorneys were quizzing physicians during medical liability actions on whether they had been required to take the oral examination. Nonetheless, these concerns alone would probably not have forced a change in the process. However, several directors were concerned that a written examination, while accurately assessing recall information and to a lesser extent interpretation, did not evaluate problem solving and judgment as well as the oral examination. This debate continued from 1980 until 1990, when the ABOto convened an educational retreat in Charlottesville, Virginia. In addition to the 25 directors of the ABOto, there were representatives from the American Board of Anesthesiology, American Board of Emergency Medicine, American Board Pediatrics, and the American Board of Surgery who served as consultants and shared their experience. As a consequence of that retreat it was decided to initiate a change in the examination process for five years, then reassess the results. The written examination became a qualifying examination with passage required prior to being allowed to sit for the oral examination. The written and oral examinations' scores were no longer combined; a candidate was required to pass both the written and, independently, the oral examination in order to become certified.

Current Examination Process

The written examination administered by the ABOto consists of 300 multiple-choice questions developed by a task force of 36 specially chosen and trained otolaryngologists who serve for two three-year terms. Many of these individuals go on to become guest examiners and directors.

Each question goes through a six-step process. Psychometricians from the American College Testing (Iowa City) assist in the process. Each question is carefully checked for content, grammar and wording to be certain that no ambiguity exists. As a final step the examination committee of the board (all of whom are directors) reviews each test question, assigns questions to a classification, and considers relevance and clinical applicability. These directors have the authority to reject any question not considered appropriate. The examination is then constructed using questions chosen by the examination committee to cover all facets of the specialty.

Seventy-five questions are chosen which had previously been used in a given year; 75 are chosen which were used previously in a different year, and 75 new questions are chosen which have been previously "field tested." These 225 questions are those on which the grade is based. Seventy-five additional new questions are "field tested" and are scored but not counted in the grade assigned to the candidate. Performance on these field-tested questions allows the examination committee to validate further the quality and reliability of the individual questions. By comparing the scores of current candidates with those obtained in the two previous years, a comparison can be made of the knowledge acquisition of the current group with each of the two previous groups (test equating). This process serves to further validate the examination process, and allows the committee responsible for setting the passing score to adjust it upward or downward based on these comparisons. In fact, the correlations have been so consistent over the years that adjustments are rarely made; when adjustments have been made, they have not exceeded one-tenth of a point.

The written examination, given to all candidates in the fall in Chicago, is taken by approximately 350 candidates in two four-hour sessions on one day. The pass rate on the written examination has been roughly 85 percent for the past five years.

The oral examination, given to all who successfully complete the written examination, consists of 16 protocols developed by directors, associate examiners, and experienced guest examiners. These protocols are divided into four categories: Facial plastic and reconstructive surgery, general otolaryngology, head and neck surgery, and otology/neurotology. One hour (50 minutes of direct questioning) is allotted to each of these categories. The examiner is chosen for this area based on demonstrated expertise in the subspecialty area. Within each subspecialty category there are in turn four protocols, one each devoted to diagnosis, treatment, emergency management, and complications. Protocols are derived from actual cases. The examination committee reviews each protocol for accuracy, content and relevance. Each consists of a brief history, physical findings, laboratory and radiological results. Candidates request information from the examiner as they proceed through the case. The amount of information provided to the candidate depends on the protocol. On the diagnostic protocols little written information is provided; the candidate is expected to elicit a complete history, perform a complete physical examination, order appropriate laboratory or radiological tests, formulate a differential diagnosis, and provide management. On the treatment protocols, more written information is provided and the focus is on management. The emergency treatment and complication protocols focus on those areas.

Standardization of each protocol is achieved by providing examiners the appropriate line of questioning *with answers* listed, thus preventing individual examiner bias from influencing scoring of cases in which several options are acceptable. Additionally, the protocols are thoroughly reviewed by all examiners the night before the examination. This allows full discussion by the group to obtain consensus on protocol content, questions, and expected answers.

In some protocols, the laboratory and radiological results are provided, but in most only after the candidate requests them. Radiographs, scans, and pathologic specimens are provided to the candidates.

Examiners are instructed to use all four protocols to give the candidates as many cases as possible and to afford the candidates a broader exposure upon which to base the scores. Examiners are not allowed to examine candidates known to them.

Scores are given on each protocol in recall, interpretation, and problem solving, and are combined across protocols into three overall scores for each subspecialty area. Examiners record scores on a card at the end of each one-hour session, and the cards are collected at the end of each half-day session. The scores for all four subspecialty areas are recorded, tallied, and averaged to arrive at a final score.

Scoring is based on a 12-point scale as follows: 1, 2, and 3 = failure; 4, 5, 6 = marginal; 7, 8, 9 = good, and 10, 11, 12 = outstanding. Since 6.8 to 7 is the usual passing range, one or more scores below this level places the candidate in danger of failing. For example, one failing, two marginal, and one good score would cause the candidate to fail; whereas two good and two high marginal would probably result in a passing score.

In order to minimize examiner variability, examiner training sessions are held every year on the day prior to the examination. All examiners, including board directors, attend a one or a one-half day session devoted to examination administration in which examination techniques and pitfalls to avoid are discussed using lectures, demonstrations, and videotapes. The examiners also practice grading an observed, simulated examination. Individual scores are compared in group sessions with senior examiners explaining scoring rules. All returning examiners receive data on their previous year's scoring of candidates, comparisons with other examiners, and final candidate grades. These training exercises serve as a fairly effective behavioral modifier.

Results

As with the written examination, the oral examination results in a passing rate in the 85 percent range; the overall passing rate, therefore, is about 70 percent of initial candidates.

After the ABOto instituted the requirement that all candidates pass both the written and oral examinations, an interesting finding emerged when assessing those candidates who received high scores on the written examination and would, therefore, have previously been certified without an oral examination: In the 1991/1992 examination cycle, twenty-three (23) candidates who would have been certified based on high written scores alone failed the oral examination; in 1992/1993, nineteen (19); and in 1993/1994, twenty-seven (27).

Thus, in the three examination cycles from 1991 through 1994, sixty-nine candidates who would have been certified by the previous examination method now failed the oral examination. The exact significance of this finding is uncertain, but one might conclude that a high score on a written examination, based primarily on recall, does not necessarily translate into high scores on an oral examination assessing interpretation or problem-solving skills. This is no surprise to the boards who have felt for many years that an oral examination is required to assess a candidate's judgment and problem-solving ability, but the impact of this finding on internal medicine, pediatrics, or other boards who certify based solely on a written examination is at this time uncertain.

A number of issues related to the oral examination appeared, perhaps not unexpectedly, beginning with the 1991/1992 cycle. For example, reflecting the greater number of candidates (nearly triple) being tested, there was a parallel shift to a larger number of inexperienced examiners. Prior to 1991, most candidates had been examined by two or three board directors during their four examination sessions. With the change, most candidates are examined by only one director and three non-director guest examiners. This lack of experienced examiners is being corrected with the introduction of thirty-six associate board examiners, all of whom have examined at least three times; currently, of roughly one hundred examiners, sixty are experienced (examined three or four times), and half the remaining forty examiners have examined at least once before.

A second change in the examination process was a doubling of the protocols. It is theoretically possible that the abrupt increase in the number of protocols could have affected their quality, but the same rigorous standards for design and screening protocols have been applied.

A third change involved the subcategories of the examination process. In previous years, each examiner was expected to present protocols to the candidates from the subspecialties of facial plastic surgery, general otolaryngology, head and neck surgery, and otology. With the new examination process, however, an expert in each of these subspecialties presents the candidate with four protocols in the subspecialty of their expertise. It is possible that a subspecialist might unconsciously hold a candidate to a higher standard in the area of their expertise than in an area of less familiarity.

The shift to a step-wise sequence of qualifying and certifying examinations was accomplished without changing the pass/fail cutoff score. In retrospect, it may have been wise, in light of the changes described above, to create a means to evaluate inter-examiner variability. In reviewing the patterns of examination scores, there are occasional differences in scoring by experienced versus inexperienced examiners, on both high and low scores for both examiner groups. Extreme examples would be sufficient to affect the pass/fail decision. Of course, such differences may have been the result of a major difference in competence from one subspecialty area to another, and the divergent scores may have been entirely valid. A careful study of this variability by the board's examination committee and psychometricians has documented no clear pattern, however, and no change in scoring procedures has been recommended.

The correlation between written examination scores and oral examination scores, and longitudinal comparisons of certification results both warrant additional comment. Each year the ABOto analyzes the correlation between the results for the written examination and those of the oral examination. There appears to be a high correlation between performance on the written examination and on the oral examination. Nonetheless, we have carefully avoided claims that the correlation between examination formats is sufficiently high to warrant elimination of one examination (presumably the oral) and by implication suggest that the oral examination may be unnecessary. There is still no satisfactory explanation as to why those who would have been certified based on high written scores failed the oral examination, unless the oral examination is measuring abilities not measured by the written examination, or the oral examination process is producing instances of inappropriate stringency (failure) on the basis of its inherently subjective nature.

Analysis of the longitudinal outcomes of the oral examination for certification is also required. If the oral examination provides an accurate assessment of a candidate's judgment and problem-solving ability, then the cost in time and dollars required to give the oral examination to all candidates is justified. This would be particularly true if the oral examination could identify individual specialists whose practice would be dangerous because of deficiencies in judgment and problem-solving ability. Unfortunately, however, the assumption that the oral examination can accomplish this task more effectively than the written examination does not hold up under careful scrutiny of the eventual outcomes in our specialty. Candidates do not receive additional training after they have failed the certification process. They return to their daily practice and, while a few read and attend courses, it is unlikely that they will be exposed to any additional training likely to enhance their judgment or problem-solving ability. When these candidates return for reexamination a second, third, or fourth time, most are eventually successful and achieve certification. Indeed, a recent analysis of several cohorts of candidates indicated that eventually between 95 percent and 97 percent of U.S. and Canadian medical school graduates ultimately achieve certification by the American Board of Otolaryngology. It is likely that these individuals have studied more intensely and have become strongly motivated by their previous failure. Armed with an expanded fund of knowledge, and perhaps more careful about mannerisms, dress, and interpersonal interactions with examiners, or perhaps simply because "practice makes perfect," these candidates are able to achieve a passing score. They demonstrate the ability to pass successfully through a screening mechanism which involves the examiners' perception of their professionalism, attitude, confidence, and other factors. It might be possible for a candidate to experience just the wrong combination of protocol topics and examiners on one occasion, resulting in an unsuccessful outcome, but have the "right" combination of topics and examiners on another occasion, and pass. There is also the possibility that a candidate could have "a bad day." It is not inconceivable that such factors as nervousness, insomnia, respiratory infection, indigestion, or stresses at home might play a role in examination failure.

Based on the observations of the last decade, it is impossible to draw more firm conclusions about the oral examination of the American Board of Otolaryngology. We are convinced that the oral examination process has merit, and we are committed to offering and improving the oral examination. In the last analysis, however, we must admit that we cannot unequivocally state that an oral examination is absolutely necessary to provide certification of capable practitioners.

Recent Changes in the Obstetrics and Gynecology Oral Examination

Albert B. Gerbie, M.D.
William Droegemueller, M.D.
The American Board of Obstetrics and Gynecology

In 1978 the evaluation committee of the American Board of Obstetrics and Gynecology (ABOG) recommended that the board adopt a definition of competence that a candidate should obtain in order to be certified as a diplomate: "A diplomate of The American Board of Obstetrics and Gynecology is a medical specialist who has demonstrated a level of competence which allows the individual to serve as a consultant to non-obstetrician/gynecologists in their community." (See Figure 1)

Figure 1. Definition of Obstetrician-Gynecologist

Obstetrician-gynecologists are physicians who, by virtue of satisfactory completion of a defined course of graduate medical education and appropriate certification, possess special knowledge, skills, and professional capability in the medical and surgical care of the female reproductive system and associated disorders, that it distinguishes them from other physicians and enables them to serve as consultants to other physicians and as primary physicians for women.

Over the years of practice, each obstetrician-gynecologist builds on this broad base of knowledge and skills and may develop a unique type of practice and changing professional focus. Such diversity contributes to high quality health care for women.

For 65 years the American Board of Obstetrics and Gynecology has employed a three-component process for certification: A written examination, a two-year practice requirement, and an oral examination. The written examination is the most effective way to examine for cognitive information; however, in our view the oral examination best emphasizes behavioral aspects of a candidate's independent practice. The oral examination evaluates the candidate's competence for solving clinical problems in obstetrics and gynecology and his or her ability to act as a consultant to the non-obstetrician/gynecologist.

ABOG continually tries to improve our examinations in pursuit of our goal to document competence. As part of this dynamic process, the board has called upon educational consultants on many occasions: Drs. Charles Dohner and Harold Levine in 1976; Dr. John Lloyd in 1980; Drs. Charles Dohner and Harold Levine in 1981; and Drs. Charles Dohner and Benson Munger in 1987. In such formal reviews the various consultants observed the oral certifying examinations and presented recommendations to the board. As a result of these consultations and also reflecting our own continuous internal review, many changes have been put in place over the years.

1. The orientation for both the new and old examiners was made more specific.
2. The examiner fatigue factor was addressed by decreasing the number of examining sessions per examiner from three a day to two.
3. The examination itself was lengthened from two to three hours, and structured case histories were introduced as part of the examination.
4. Senior examiners were assigned to the candidates' lounges to relieve the anxiety of the candidates waiting to be examined.
5. The addition of an initial hour (now half-hour), during which the candidate reviews two-by-two projection slides and five microscopic slides. The candidate is alone during this time, giving him or her a chance to release tension in a "cooling off" period.

A new emphasis has been placed on the practice experience; approximately half of the oral exam questions are now derived from the candidates' own case lists, lists derived from care rendered over one to two years, with experience as the constant and time the variable. The other half of the examination consists of hypothetical questions about patient management based upon structured clinical cases and slides selected by the board.

In the past, individual examiners asked questions covering the breadth and depth of the entire specialty. A recent change was made, however, in the rotation of examiners which significantly alters this picture. An examiner is now assigned specifically to the domains of obstetrics, gynecology, or outpatient/primary care. The examiner now tests each candidate on clinical problems in the specific area assigned using obstetric, gynecologic, or office practice 35 mm slides, structured cases, and the candidate's case list as guides for discussion.

It is pertinent to review precisely how the 35 mm slides are used. There are approximately five slides for each clinical domain. The examiners are instructed that these are not for identification per se, but rather are to be used as patient management problems or mini-CPCs.

Figure 2. "Check List" for Evaluating a Candidate

I. Ability to approach patient management problems.
   A. Elicits data in an organized fashion.
   B. Evaluates data and combinations of data.
   C. Formulates differential diagnosis—logical: common/rare.
   D. Performs no harmful test or procedure.
   E. Familiar with diagnostic and therapeutic procedures.
      1. Indications
      2. Contraindications
      3. Complications
      4. Alternative procedures
   F. Overall logical approach and treatment.

II. Affect—examinee's attitude toward problem. (Not a measure of hostility in relation to examiner but approach in handling the patient.)

III. Recall and specific interpretation. (Relatively few questions.)

IV. State of the examinee—anxiety, language problems.

The examiner must recognize which questions only elicit information demonstrated by "recall" and those questions which are more sophisticated and require the examinee to synthesize a judgment based on information he has elicited.

Ten different sets of slides are used, permitting the slides to be changed every half-day over the five days of an examination period. In obstetrics the slides might include, for example, fetal monitor strips, a genetics pedigree, and ultrasound delineation of fetal anomalies. In the gynecology section the slides could encompass a photograph of retroperitoneal anatomy, colposcopy photos, or operative photographs of, for example, a uterine prolapse, while in office practice/primary care, features of endocrinopathy, a vulvar rash, an abnormal mammogram, and slides of vaginal discharge might be illustrated. Utilizing the same category of slides for each candidate helps to establish uniformity from candidate to candidate.

For viewing purposes, an easel with dry-erase pens is used rather than a projection screen. The clinical problem under discussion is projected onto the easel. With the dry-erase pen the candidate can draw on the easel to demonstrate where to, for example, excise tissue, or to demonstrate knowledge of operative anatomy, or to document understanding of monitor strips. Interaction with the examiner improves the quality of the process. These slides and the clinical cases allow the board to assess a variety of clinical skills, including the interpretation of labor curves, fetal monitor strips, ultrasounds, colposcopy, laparoscopy, amniocentesis, karyotypes, laboratory results, genetic counseling, contraception counseling, menopause management, and primary/preventive care.

In any given examination session, 225 examiners are utilized, divided into 70 teams of three examiners. The teams are reconstituted each day. During the five days of examination, 350 teams examine approximately 1,200 candidates. The teams meet at the end of each examining session and independently grade the candidates. This process has resulted in a remarkably uniform pass rate over the past five years analyzed for each examination year in Tables 1 to 3. The percentage of passes by year of examination administration is found in Table 1, documenting a range of pass rates between 83 percent and 87 percent for the oral exam. Since the recent changes in the examination process as outlined above, the pass rates have been 86 or 87 percent.

Table 1. American Board of Obstetrics & Gynecology Oral Examination Pass Rates

Year	Total Examined	Pass Rate (#) %
1990	1298	(1100) 85
1991	1270	(1053) 83
1992	1330	(1148) 86
1993	1186	(1032) 87
1994	1375	(1193) 87

A further analysis of pass rates by specific topical area is in Table 2. There is no difference in the pass/fail rates in the specific areas of examination. Table 3 illustrates the fact that the particular day of the examination has no significant impact on pass/fail rates.

Table 2. Pass/Fail Rate by Area of Examination				
Year	**Total Examined**	**Ob**	**Gyn**	**Off**
1994	1375	1183 (86%)	1196 (87%)	1196 (87%)
1993	1186	1032 (87%)	1020 (86%)	1032 (87%)

Table 3. 1994 Pass Rate on Oral Examination by Day of Administration				
Monday	**Tuesday**	**Wednesday**	**Thursday**	**Friday**
274 (86%)	**278 (86%)**	**270 (87%)**	**283 (86%)**	**270 (89%)**

In summary, the evaluation committee of the American Board of Obstetrics and Gynecology has made several recent modifications in the oral examination process. These changes have been well received by both candidates and examiners. The board believes the consistency of the data is the result of the changes we have initiated over the past 15 years.

Suggested Reading

1. Arndt CB, Guly UMV, McManus IC. Preclinical anxiety: the stress associated with *viva voce* examination. *Med Educ* 1986;20:274-80.

2. Eagle CJ, Martineau R, Hamilton K. The oral examination in anaesthetic resident evaluation. *Can J Anaesth* 1993;40:947-53.

3. McDermott JF Jr, Tanguay PE, Scheiber SC, et al. Reliability of the Part II board certification examination in psychiatry: interexaminer consistency. *Am J Psychiatry* 1991;148:1672-4.

4. McDermott JF Jr, Tanguay PE, Scheiber SC, et al. Reliability of the Part II board certification examination in psychiatry: examination stability. *Am J Psychiatry* 1993;150:1077-80.

5. Solomon DJ, Reinhart MA, Bridgham RG, et al. An assessment of an oral examination format for evaluating clinical competence in emergency medicine. *Acad Med* 1990;65(S9);S43-4.

Assumptions in Scoring Oral Examinations

Philip G. Bashook, Ed.D.
American Board of Medical Specialties

In 1974, Steven Cahn, a philosopher at the University of Vermont, was invited to offer his comments on the board examinations used to certify physicians. His remarks were published in the *American Journal of Medicine*; they are most appropriate for today's discussion. He said,

> "The standard of excellence must be decided. Those who meet it pass, those who do not fail. If a board cannot decide the standard of excellence, it is unclear what its examination is testing, apart from the relative standing of those taking the test at any one time."[1]

Clearly, every certifying board has two fundamental decisions to make:

1. Establish the standard for certification of candidates.
2. Decide who gets certified.

Ultimately, every applicant to the board either is or is not certified; there is no middle ground. Even those applicants who repeatedly fail and reapply eventually must either be certified or not at the discretion of the board. The point of a yes/no certification decision by the board is stressed here because it is essential in appreciating the assumptions in scoring oral examinations.

There are, of course, many other actions made by the board leading to each of these fundamental decisions. For example, among the 24 ABMS Member Boards 15 boards use written examinations to qualify candidates and standardized oral examinations as the final certifying examination. Objectivity, fairness, properly sampled topics and cases, test design, trained examiners, agreed upon board standards, are among the carefully planned factors that affect the quality of oral examinations and influence a board's certification decisions.

With this background in mind, there are four assumptions in scoring oral examinations which are pivotal to decisions about who becomes board certified. Each will be mentioned briefly and then elaborated upon. The assumptions are phrased as questions to help stimulate discussion.

1. **What to do about marginal candidates?**
2. **Which is better, pass/fail scoring or rating scales?**
3. **How should scores from subtests be combined to make a pass/fail decision?**
4. **What effect does the interaction between candidates, examiners, and cases have on the quality of scores?**

Let us begin by considering the first assumption, **What to do about marginal candidates?**

Consistent with the philosophical position of Dr. Cahn, *there is no such thing as a marginal candidate; however, there may be marginal data about a candidate which was collected during the oral examination.* If the data collected about the candidate during an oral examination appears to be inconclusive for a yes/no decision, the board must decide whether to certify the candidate or gather more data on the candidate's abilities. There are two straightforward tasks a board may wish to consider to avoid encountering the problem of "marginal data about a candidate."

The first task in planning future exams is to review the current exam by asking: Is the exam fair? Do the candidate scores accurately reflect candidate performance? Is there a sufficient number of cases or should more cases be used to assure sufficient exam data for potential candidates who generate marginal data? Are the examiners asking appropriate questions to assess the thinking abilities of the candidates or does the questioning only assess recall and memory?

The second task is to plan to incorporate into future examination schedules time for reexamining candidates, or plan examinations with the expectation candidates from prior exams will be completing additional sessions. The former is preferred due to security issues when candidates have days or months between examination subtests. The following questions are offered as a guide: Are candidates informed before they arrive for the oral examination that their exam time may be extended because additional performance data may be needed? Does the oral examination schedule include open slots to allow for further testing of some candidates? Are candidates' performance scores reviewed before discharging candidates from the exam and in time to allow further testing?

In summary, there are no marginal candidates, only marginal exam data about candidates which hinders making pass/fail decisions.

The second assumption to be addressed is, **Which is better, pass/fail scoring or rating scales?**

Both have advantages and disadvantages and both are useful for different reasons. The simplest answer is to use both. Table 1 summarizes the advantages and disadvantages of pass/fail scoring.

Table 1. Pass/Fail Scoring

Advantages

1. The examiners who make pass/fail decisions are most knowledgeable about the candidate's performance because they asked the questions and directly grade candidates.
2. Pass/fail scoring eliminates the need for post-exam discussions about passing candidates.
3. Scoring formulae can be simplified for exam subtests and the overall exam.

Disadvantages

1. Extensive examiner training is required.
2. When examiners disagree there may be insufficient data to reconcile pass/fail recommendations.
3. One examiner can decide the fate of a candidate unless scoring rules negate this possibility.
4. Potentially important data about candidates with marginal data is not available using only pass/fail scoring.

Table 2 summarizes the advantages and disadvantages of using rating scales.

Table 2. Rating Scales

Advantages

1. Fine distinctions in case performance can be recorded by examiners.
2. Individual subtest scores can be combined to derive a final pass/fail score.
3. Various statistical analyzes can be applied to rating scales which are not possible with pass/fail scoring.

Disadvantages

1. Extensive examiner training is required.
2. Rating scales may be interpreted differently by different examiners (i.e., examiners frequently do not use end-points on rating scales; some examiners are inconsistent in applying scaling rules; and examiners often differ in how they define individual scale point values.
3. Decisions about passing a candidate usually are not made by the examiner testing the candidate but by a committee interpreting examiner(s) reports or through scoring algorithms.
4. Rating scale points are assumed to be one unit apart for statistical calculations but are rarely verified, thus generating potentially inaccurate scoring statistics.

Often, rating scales are designed in three segments: Clearly passing scores (e.g., 7-10), clearly failing scores (e.g., 1-4), and conditional or marginal passing scores (e.g., 5-6). In reality these are three point scales in which the examiner has the leeway to add intermediate scale points. Post-exam statistical analyses assume that these intermediate scale points are distinct and equivalent to the broadly defined segments separating passing and failing performance. However, this assumption is not often verified.

In summary, both rating scales and pass/fail scoring are useful for oral examinations especially in evaluating the performance data for candidates who generate marginal data.

The third important assumption in scoring oral exams is, **How should scores from subtests be combined to make a pass/fail decision?** The scoring rules for combining subtest scores should be based upon the conditions set forth in the examination blueprint. Livingston and Zieky describe the commonly used scoring algorithms.[2] For example, it is common to develop an exam blueprint which defines a number of exam subsections or subtests. Each subtest is considered an essential component of the overall test and must be passed. In medical specialty oral exams it is common to group the clinical cases into disciplines of the specialty, patient characteristics, or treatment opportunities (e.g., emergency care situations, patients presenting with an acute phase of a chronic illness, diagnosis and treatment of patients from a specific age group, treatment of patients with complex multi-diseases, trauma care). When exam sessions are constructed to correspond to the case groupings, each becomes an oral exam subtest. If candidates must pass all subtests to pass the oral exam then scores on each subtest are treated as either pass or fail and candidates who pass all subtests pass, those who fail one or more subtests fail overall. Alternatively, the exam blueprint will sometimes define clusters of subtests required to be passed. In this case the subtest scores are grouped for each cluster and pass/fail decisions made per cluster. Candidates may fail one or more subtests in a cluster and still pass the overall test. If the combining of subtest scores does not conform to the exam blueprint, then there is a question of the exam's validity. This scoring approach would be considered *criterion-referenced or domain-referenced scoring*. It can create difficulties in exam design and analysis when cases overlap subtests resulting in moderate correlations between subtest scores.

On the other hand, the exam blueprint might be constructed so that the number of cases are defined for each domain but cases are mixed among exam sessions and no session constitutes a subtest. Each candidate, then, encounters in each session a variety of cases drawn randomly from the collection of cases in the total examination. Each exam session is a time-slot to allow sampling of cases across specialty domains. This technique is not commonly used in oral examinations, especially in the medical specialties. However, scoring such an exam could use *compensatory scoring*. In compensatory scoring, individual subtest scores (each exam session) are added together to obtain a total exam score. Exam sessions serve only to separate the test into manageable time periods and are structured according to topics in the exam blueprint. Poor performance in one session can be compensated for by superior performance in another.

A third method of combining exam subtest scores is by *grading-on-the-curve or relative performance score*. A common method is to identify first-time candidates on the exam, average their scores, and use the average to set the passing score at one or two standard deviations below it. This reference group of candidates is drawn from the current exam, not previous exams or a separate exam administration. As such, the performance on the current exam cannot be compared to previous exams, although identical cases used in both exams may be compared for raw scores. Also, setting the passing score based upon candidates who have taken the exam amounts to judging all candidates on the quality of a few, not against the board's certification standard. Comparing or equating performance on the current exam with prior exams is not possible.

It is not hard to understand how a board can set a standard of excellence for each subtest. But, why should poor performance on one subtest be allowed to be compensated for by superior performance on another? Also, why judge one candidate's performance against another by grading-on-the-curve when neither may meet the board's defined standard of excellence? To reiterate my initial point, boards decide who will be *certified* not whether a candidate ranks as excellent, marginal, or another category. Certificates are not issued with a class ranking stamped upon them.

The forth and last assumption to be discussed is, **What effect does the interaction between candidates, examiners, and cases have on the quality of scores?**

Very little research has been done on the nature of the interactions between candidates, examiners, and cases in standardized oral examinations. The psychometric attributes of each component, however, have been investigated (See Appendix III and particularly papers by Barnes and Pressy, Butzin et al, Colton and Peterson, Kelly et al, Lindsey, Lunz and Stahl, Maatsch et al, McDermott et al, McGuire, Meskauskas, Muzzin and Hart, Newble et al, Raymond, Solomon et al, Trimble, Waugh and Moyse, Wilson et al, Yange and Laube). Most studies have looked at *un-standardized* exams for college students, graduate students, medical students, and residents in training, frequently without the equivalent high-stakes consequences of certification exams. The studies assume the interactions introduce errors into the scoring equation which need statistical correction. Available research about the interactions in oral exams can be summarized in a few sentences:

1. Research on examiner questioning style suggests that most examiners ask recall or memory questions.[3, 4]
2. A number of studies about candidates' personality characteristics, candidate's anxiety, and communication style during the exam suggest that these factors influence examiners' decisions.[3, 5, 6, 7, 8, 9]
3. Variability in scoring by multiple examiners assessing the same candidate has been established.[10, 11, 12]
4. One study on case difficulty suggested it was a minor contributor to examiner's scoring decisions.[13]
5. No published studies report findings about the three-way interaction between candidates-examiners-cases.

It is time to focus upon the sociometrics of oral examinations. There are important questions to consider when the exam is viewed from a sociometric perspective.[14] What is known about how examiners' personal bias influencing the scoring? What about the effect of the pace of the exam? What about the influence that sequencing of cases has upon candidate's performance? Are there systematic ways to adjust scores for mis-communication by examiner and/or candidate? How long is the preferred time to examine on each case? Does exam time vary by case complexity? What is the impact on examiners' decisions when a candidate develops severe test anxiety? What happens when two examiners evaluating the same candidate have very different examining styles? Many questions, but only limited anecdotal data available to answer them.

In summary, discussed in this paper have been four assumptions about oral examinations: Marginal candidates, pass/fail vs rating scale scoring, combining subtest scores, and the paucity of sociometric research on oral examinations. The list of assumptions could easily be expanded. The four were chosen because they are common to many if not all oral examinations. I hope this paper suggests why it is important to consider carefully the underlying issues and assumptions when selecting a scoring schema.

References

1. Cahn SM. Philosophical reflections on evaluation. *Am J Med* 1974; 57:152-156.

2. Livingston SA, Zieky MJ. *Passing scores.* Princeton, NJ: Educational Testing Service 1982.

3. Evans LR, Ingersoll RW, Smith EJ. The reliability, validity, and taxonomic structure of the oral examination. *J Med Educ* 1966; 41:651-657.

4. McGuire CH. The oral examination as a measure of professional competence. *J Med Educ* 1966; 41:267-274.

5. Green EW, Evans LR, Ingersoll RW. The reactions of students in the oral examination. *J Med Educ* 1967; 42:345-349.

6. Platt JR. On maximizing the information obtained from science examinations, written and oral. *Am J Physics* 1961; 29:111-122.

7. Vassend O. Examination stress, personality and self-reported physical symptoms. *Scan J Psychology* 1988; 29:21-32.

8. Rowland-Moran PA, Burchard KW, Garb JL, Coe NPW. Influence of effective communication by surgery students on their oral examination scores. *Acad Med* 1991; 66:169-171.

9. Thomas CS, Mellsop G, Callender K, Crawshaw J, Ellis PM, Hall A, MacDonald J, Silfverskiold P, Romans-Clarkson S. The Oral Examination: A study of academic and non-academic factors. *Med Educ* 1992; 27:433-439.

10. Pokorny AD, Frazier Jr SH. An evaluation of oral examinations. *J Med Educ* 1966; 41:28-40.

11. Kelly Jr PR, Matthews JH, Schumacher CF. Analysis of the oral examination of the American Board of Anesthesiology. *J Med Educ* 1971; 46:982-988.

12. Marshall VR, Ludbrook J. The relative importance of patient and examiner variability in a test of clinical skills. *Brit J Med Educ* 1972; 6:212-217.

13. Leichner P, Sisler GC, Harper D. The clinical oral examination in psychiatry: Association between subscoring and global marks. *Can J Psychiatry* 1986; 31:750-751.

14. Remer R. Improving oral exams—an application of Morenean sociometry. *J Grp Psychotherapy, Psychodrama, and Sociometry* 1990; 43:35-42.

Statistical Methods to Improve Decision Reproducibility

Mary E. Lunz, Ph.D.
American Society of Clinical Pathologists – Board of Registry

Studies to improve examinations have produced examination blueprints,[1] consensus-based case protocols,[2] extensive training of examiners,[3,4] calibration of examiners for grading severity,[5,6] consistency of examination procedures, and structured scoring and reporting procedures.[7] Some medical specialty boards have replaced case protocols with the "chart stimulated recall" using a candidate's actual medical records,[8,9] or with the presentation of practice-based cases.

Orals are individualized examinations meant to assess cognitive skill and judgment. The examiner can pursue candidate strengths or weaknesses within the context of a case. Candidates often interact with different examiners on different cases. Thus, each oral examination is essentially a **unique test form**. It would be desirable to create some decision consistency among oral examinations so that passing the examination represents a definable standard of practice rather than an ideal in the mind of an individual examiner. Statistical methods can be used to improve consistency of pass/fail decisions within the oral examination process.

Medical specialty boards carefully structure cases and train examiners in an attempt to obtain consistency in the oral examinations. Scoring uses defined points on a rating scale that focus on levels of acceptable candidate performance. Examiners are trained, and may observe others or practice themselves in the administration of examinations. On the other hand, each candidate has a unique examination by virtue of the multiple combinations of examiners, cases, and/or tasks. Cases and examiners are rotated, for example, and examination sessions are often spread over several days. A candidate may interact with a subset of one to ten examiners from a group of 250 examiners on only six to as many as 80 standardized cases.

The ratings given to candidates by examiners comprise the data used to categorize candidates. In the ideal situation, candidates would be rated on all cases by all examiners. However, this rarely occurs; the specific interactions that constitute the unique test form are different for each candidate. As an example in Table 1, Candidate #1 interacts with Examiners X (lenient) and Y (moderate) and earns relatively high ratings on Case 2 (moderate difficulty) and Case 3 (easy). Candidate #2 interacts with Examiners Y (moderate) and Z (severe) and earns lower ratings on Case 1 (difficult) and Case 2 (moderate difficulty). Candidate #1 earns a high score on relatively easy cases from relatively lenient examiners while Candidate #2 earns a lower score on more difficult cases from relatively severe examiners. Candidate #1 passes based on a relatively easy examination. Candidate #2 fails based on a relatively difficult examination. Clearly the two candidates did not have comparable opportunities to pass. The particular combination of examiners and cases defines the difficulty of the oral examination, and each exam is different.

Table 1. Example Interactions Between Candidates, Examiners, and Cases

	Candidate #1			Candidate #2		
Case #	1	2	3	1	2	3
Examiner X		3	4			
Examiner Y		3	3	2	3	
Examiner Z				1	2	
Case Score		6	7	3	5	
	Total	13 = 81%		Total	8 = 50%	
Decision		PASS			FAIL	

Perfect Score = 16

Rating Scale
4 = excellent
3 = satisfactory
2 = below average
1 = unsatisfactory

Since there is a high probability that oral examinations will differ, such that each candidate has a unique examination experience, accounting for the differences in the exams serves to equate the examinations so that ALL candidates must demonstrate a standardized level of skill and knowledge to pass. This is parallel to golf. Each player earns a "handicap" based on his experience and previous performance. Each hole on a golf course has a "par" that is established by a board of experts based on its difficulty. If the player makes the par, he/she meets the standard for that hole; if the player does not make the par, he/she doesn't meet the standard for the hole. The same standard applies to all players. A player with a level of ability challenges a hole with an established level of difficulty. When the two meet, the result is a pass/fail decision.

Sources of Variability

Inherent in scoring a candidate's performance are two kinds of variability: Systematic variability which should be amenable to statistical analysis and control; and unsystematic variability due to unanticipated characteristics of cases, examiners, or candidates. The goal of most examinations is to classify or order candidates by ability as accurately as possible. Examiners in oral examinations, however, are human beings with different levels of education, medical practice experience, and experience with the test cases, all of which influence their performance and interactions. Examiners are, in a word, variable. Statistical techniques that quantify an examiner's approach into an overall "severity" assessment have recently been developed,[10] and can be used to equate oral examinations.

Whether standardized or practice-based, some cases are more difficult than others. Statistical analyses can also quantify cases into an overall "difficulty" assessment. As a result, both the systematic variability of examiners and of cases can be statistically accounted for. Also, differences in the difficulty of tasks within cases, e.g., diagnosis and treatment, can also be quantified and statistically accounted for.

The type of rating given by examiners is another variable. Holistic pass/fail ratings on the whole case, or analytic ratings for individual tasks within cases may be given. The definition and number of points on the rating scale also controls the examiners' ratings. A two point scale causes pass vs fail decisions by case or task within case, while a three point scale allows a pass, marginal, or fail score and a four point scale sets levels of performance such as unacceptable, poor, satisfactory or excellent. The definition of the rating scale is a variable that can also be accounted for statistically.

Unsystematic variability includes all factors that cannot be handled through careful planning of the examination. These factors often involve interpersonal interaction or individual interpretation of examiner and/or candidates. Examples of such unsystematic variability include unanticipated interpretation of standardized cases, examiners who do not follow the prescribed case protocols, and candidates who develop "uncontrollable test anxiety." Presentation of practice cases that deal with content relatively unfamiliar to the examiner may also influence the way the examiner rates a candidate's performance. Each instance, when identified, is addressed after it occurs, so reports tend to be anecdotal.

Figure 1 summarizes some of the areas of examination variability and suggests whether statistical analysis can be used to enhance control. Whether the variability is systematic or unsystematic, all aspects of the examination influence final decisions about candidates.

Figure 1. Sources of Variability in Oral or Clinical Examinations

Matrix Domain	Source of Variability*	Statistical Calibration
Examiners		
(C_j)	Reaction to candidates	not calibrate
	Personal factors/feelings	not calibrate
	Familiarity with cases	calibrate
	Specialty expertise in case	calibrate
	Sensitivity to levels performance	calibrate
	Willing to score pass/fail	calibrate
Case Skills		
(T_i)	Clarity of questions asked	not calibrate
	Data gathering	calibrate
	Diagnosis	calibrate
	Treatment/Management	calibrate
	Technical skill	calibrate
	Outcomes	calibrate
	Ethics	calibrate
Candidates		
(B_n)	Personality	not calibrate
	Articulateness	not calibrate
	Test anxiety	not calibrate
	Style of answering	not calibrate
	Reasoning ability	calibrate
	Specialty knowledge	calibrate
	Practice experience with cases	calibrate
	Skill in the specialty	calibrate

*Data is from the rating scale used by examiners to assess candidates on cases and/or tasks. (For explanation of C_j, T_i, B_n see page 104.)

Statistical Methods for Equating Oral Examination Forms

The purpose of statistical equating is to place alternate forms of the examination on a scale such that all candidates are compared to a single standard. Since each candidate's oral examination has a unique test form due to a different combination of examiners and cases, orals must be equated for candidates to have comparable opportunities to pass. Equating is accomplished through a statistical process that weights each facet of an examination form. Simply stated, a "difficult" examination earns more weight than an "easier" examination, based on several assumptions: First, alternate examination forms are meant to be comparable; second, a prescribed level of candidate ability must be demonstrated to pass; and third, the most able candidates should earn the highest ability estimate regardless of the examiners and cases in their examination.

Facets Model

The facets model was developed from the principles of the Rasch item response theory (IRT) model[11] by Linacre.[10] The basic premise of Rasch model analysis is that the most able candidate should achieve the highest ability estimate, regardless of the particular examiners and cases presented in his/her examination. See Figure 3 (page 104) for the mathematical probability equation used in the facets model. If all examiners could rate all candidates on all cases or tasks, it would be unnecessary to equate examinations; however, some examiners and cases are usually distributed among candidates, and unique examinations are provided, as already noted, for each candidate.

Results of Equating

To illustrate the value of calibrating and statistically equating examinations, data are drawn from an oral examination which included, for each candidate, six standardized cases, three cases with one examiner and three cases with another. A four point rating scale (0, 1, 2, 3) was used. One holistic rating per case was given. Ratings were summed across cases, for a maximum score of eighteen (18). Candidate examinations were calibrated using the facets model.[10] The candidate ability estimates were then translated to a scale with 400 as the pass point. The variability of the individual oral examinations with different combinations of examiners and cases and the value of calibrations is shown in Figure 2 for three unique test forms. The scoring is done first by calibrating both the examiners and cases, then equating and scaling the candidates' scores.[12]

Figure 2. Demonstration of Oral Examination Equating

Candidates	Examiner	Examiner Difficulty Calibration	Cases	Case Difficulty Calibration	Candidate Ratings
			2	Medium	2
A	15	Medium	3	Medium	2
			10	Medium	2
			6	Hard	1
	33	Medium	9	Medium	2
			4	Easy	3
			2	Medium	2
B	17	Severe	3	Medium	1
			5	Medium	2
			8	Hard	1
	13	Severe	12	Hard	1
			6	Hard	1
			4	Easy	3
C	2	Lenient	11	Easy	2
			1	Easy	3
			7	Medium	2
	3	Lenient	9	Medium	1
			10	Medium	1

Candidate A's oral examination was of moderate difficulty, with two examiners calibrated as medium in severity and a mix of six cases with an average of medium difficulty. Candidate A earned a score of 12 points on the six cases and a weighted and scaled score, after equating, of 420, a pass. This candidate had moderately difficult cases and examiners. Candidate B's oral examination included examiners who graded severely on difficult cases. Candidate B earned a score of 8 points on the six cases which, after equating, became a 409 scaled score, a pass. The candidate probably would have failed without the equating that weighted the difficulty of the cases and severity of the examiners. Candidate C's oral examination was relatively easy including lenient examiners and easy cases. Candidate C earned a score of 12 and an equated score of 370, a fail. The candidate may have passed instead of failing on the easy exam without weighting and equating the examination.

Discussion

Medical specialty boards carefully structure cases and train examiners in an attempt to standardize the oral examination. Scoring uses defined points on a rating scale. However, because cases and examiners are rotated, each candidate takes a unique examination, introducing systematic as well as unsystematic variability. The sources of variability can be defined, but cannot be controlled adequately through practice or training of examiners. Statistical calibration and equating of cases and examiners is one method of correcting much of the systematic variability. Through statistical equating, candidate ability estimates are weighted for differences in oral examination forms, and compared to established standards. Decisions are reproducible, even if the examiners and cases are altered.

Assessing cases and examiners using calibrations is similar to "key validation" in written examinations. Calibrating case difficulty can be validated by obtaining data about the case content specificity, clinical challenge, number of decision points and difficulty. Examiner calibrations can be validated with data on examiner's familiarity with the case, experience with the specific case problem, expectations for candidate performance, and attitude toward making pass/fail decisions. The statistical equating process can identify a substantial amount of variability among oral examinations forms and serves to adjust systematic variability in the exam. It also enhances the importance of input from examiners and adds a level of statistical precision to the pass/fail decisions made from oral examinations. The principles of test equating are applicable to most oral and clinical testing formats.

Statistical analysis is an objective method of "leveling the playing field." Using statistical techniques of this type, we can begin to understand the interactive structure of the oral examination process and how the oral examination facets work together to make unique test forms for individual candidates. The impact of measurement error becomes more obvious. When measurement error is decreased there is higher confidence in the accuracy of the pass/fail decisions being made and certification boards are in a better position to defend the examination results and the examination process. Equating allows the board to set the pass/fail standard, not rely upon each individual examiner, so all candidates in fact have a comparable opportunity to pass, after the differences have been accounted for statistically in the unique test forms.

As in golf, regardless of the unique test form encountered (golf course), the candidates have the same opportunity to make "par" (pass) the exam.

Figure 3. Mathematical Probability Equation

The facets model for this analysis is

$$\log (P_{nijk}/P_{nijk-1}) = (B_n - C_j - D_i - F_k)$$

in which:

P_{nijk} = the probability of candidate n being given grade k by examiner j on case i (correct).
P_{nijk-1} = the probability of candidate n being given grade k-1 by examiner j on case 1 (incorrect).

B_n = ability of candidate n
C_j = severity of examiner j
D_i = difficulty of case i
F_k = difficulty of earning step k on task

The mathematical derivation of this model appears in Linacre (1993).

Calibrations are calculated from the sum of all ratings. Case difficulty calibrations are calibrated from all ratings given to all candidates by all examiners. Examiner severity calibrations are calculated from all ratings given by the examiner across candidates and cases examined. Since each candidate takes a unique oral examination, the summative calibrations are used to equate oral examinations. This basic model is applicable to most examination formats.

References

1. Krome RL, Wagner DK, Munger BS. Standardized Oral Examinations. In Lloyd JS (Ed.) *Oral Examinations in Medical Specialty Board Certification,* Evanston, IL: American Board of Medical Specialties, 1983; pp. 25-53.

2. Mindell ER. Standardization of Oral Examinations. In Lloyd JS (Ed.) *Oral Examinations in Medical Specialty Board Certification,* Evanston, IL: American Board of Medical Specialties, 1983; pp. 55-61.

3. Stevens WC. Training of oral examiners: The oral examination workshop of the American Board of Anesthesiology. In Lloyd JS (Ed.) *Oral Examinations in Medical Specialty Board Certification,* Evanston, IL: American Board of Medical Specialties, 1983; pp. 73-78.

4. Trier WC. Oral Examiner Training by the American Board of Plastic Surgery. In Lloyd JS (Ed.) *Oral Examinations in Medical Specialty Board Certification,* Evanston, IL: American Board of Medical Specialties, 1983; pp. 79-82.

5. Lunz ME, Stahl JA. Judge consistency and severity across grading periods. *Eval and the Hlth Prof,* 1990; 13:425-444.

6. Lunz ME, Stahl JA. Impact of examiners on candidate scores: an introduction to the use of multifacet Rasch model analysis for oral examinations. *Teachg and Learng Med* 1993; 5:174-181.

7. Butzin DW, Finberg L, Brownlee RD, Guerin RO. A study of the grading process used in the American Board of Pediatrics' oral examination. In Lloyd JS (Ed.) *Oral Examinations in Medical Specialty Board Certification,* Evanston, IL: American Board of Medical Specialties, 1983 pp. 101-109.

8. Neale HW, Puckett CL. Clinical Case Review. In Mancall EL and Bashook PG (Eds.) *Recertification: New evaluation methods and strategies.* Evanston, IL: American Board of Medical Specialties, 1994 pp. 57-62

9. Munger B. Oral examinations. In Mancall EL and Bashook PG (Eds.) *Recertification: New evaluation methods and strategies.* Evanston, IL: American Board of Medical Specialties, 1994 pp. 39-42.

10. Linacre JM. *FACETS,* a computer program for analysis of examinations with multiple facets. Chicago: Mesa Press, 1993.

11. Rasch G. *Probabilistic models for some intelligence and attainment tests.* Chicago: University of Chicago Press, 1960/1980.

12. Lunz ME, Stahl JA, Wright BD. Interjudge reliability and decision reproducibility. *Educ Psychol Meas,* 1994; 54:4, 913-915.

Discussion

Dr. Norman Hertz (California Department of Consumer Affairs): My question relates to using the compensatory scoring versus a non-compensatory scoring model. The use of a non-compensatory model will invariably depress the passing percentage. It is my understanding that to support such a model the different content areas in the blueprint should be statistically independent and be able to measure the content with such a very high degree of specificity that you can be assured that the area is being well measured. On the other hand, a compensatory model allows you some slack in your assumptions about the different content areas. So my question again is, how supportable is a non-compensatory model?

Dr. Philip G. Bashook (American Board of Medical Specialties): My answer is really the conceptual answer. If you have defined those domains separately, then you should show some statistical separation between them. If you are sampling from each domain in such a way that you have a sufficient number of cases to be able to have a representative sample, you should be able to establish that that area is acceptable or unacceptable. If you are then willing to allow an individual to marginally pass that area, if you'd like to use that term, and allow that to be adjusted, you are changing the basic assumption of your test.

Dr. Mary E. Lunz (Board of Registry, American Society of Clinical Pathologists): I just wanted to say that when you construct parts of an examination, you actually have extensive control over the exam difficulty. In determining how difficult the exam will be, in some ways determines how many individuals will pass. I think it is easy to forget that the difficulty factor is always there underlying every part of any examination and obviously influencing pass/fail decisions.

Dr. Bashook: I wanted to open the door to anybody in the audience, as well as the panel, to respond to these questions. When would you recommend not using an oral exam? What separates using it from not using it? Secondly, to Dr. Scheiber, when would you not recommend using live patients?

Dr. Stephen C. Scheiber (American Board of Psychiatry & Neurology): The board's oral exam has been criticized because it does not give enough time for candidates, only a half-hour is available, for interviewing a patient. At least that was the previous criticism. As long as the patient-doctor interaction is valued, the exam picks up on cues, and is thorough, and as long as the two fields that we represent, psychiatry and neurology, continue to feel strongly about assessing candidates using real patients, I think we are committed to using real patients. At the other end of the scale is the problem of logistics for the examination. It certainly is becoming increasingly difficult, since most exams are still held in hospital settings.

Dr. Mancall: Is there anybody from Pediatrics or Medicine who wants to comment about the logistical issue?

Dr. Robert O. Guerin (American Board of Pediatrics): I think the board dropped the oral examination for reasons other than logistics, or at least reasons beyond logistics had greater priority. The number of candidates has increased fairly significantly, nearly doubled, since dropping the oral, so the problem would be even greater in 1995 than before. The issue is not one of cost alone. One of the board examiners reminded me after the session this morning that the oral exam took at least thirty days each year out of an examiner's life. The board had 200 examiners for the oral exams, and today the board would probably need more than double that number, more like an exponential growth. With an increase in the number of examiners there is a need to increase the number of examinees on learning status and on training status. At some point, the whole process might just break down. It's unaffordable, both in terms of physician time and of training time. It's a difficult question to address. At what point is it necessary to say that a very reliable, valid examination cannot be used because of the logistic problems? A sad situation, unfortunately. Some of the important exam components may be shifted as assessments in the training programs where there is more control, for example, and more ability to investi-gate communication skills, psychomotor skills and such.

Dr. Bernard-M. Lefevbre (Royal College of Physicians and Surgeons of Canada): The first question about when to drop the oral examination I would answer, because of cost. Right now the Royal College charges candidates for the entire examination, a complete examination, $2,000 a year, Canadian. The College does not expend additional money only the candidates' fees. The second question is about the use of live patients. When the Royal College uses live patients, one of the problems is we cannot do what Dr. Lunz was saying, decide on the pass/fail standard. It has to be the individual examiners who decide because they are dealing with a particular patient for a particular candidate. The other question is the review mechanism. We receive many requests for reviews when live patients are used on the examination. I would like to give you an anecdote about reviewing performance with live patients. A patient, who was part of the examination in Internal Medicine, happened to have a total hip prosthesis which dislocated during the examination. The exam experience was quite distressing for the candidate *and* the examiner.

Dr. Kerry Hampshire (American Board of Clinical Neuropsychology): Given the complexity and the delicacies of the oral examinations, I wonder if panel members could comment about the selection of the examiners. How long do you retain an examiner? How long are the appointments and to what degree is the selection of non-university, that is private practice-based clinicians, important for assembling examining teams?

Dr. Francis P. Hughes (American Board of Anesthesiology): I touched on that briefly in my remarks. The board receives nominations for examiners from a variety of sources. An individual could self-nominate, or they could be nominated by another diplomate of the board, perhaps an associate examiner. The board looks carefully at the nominations, asks associate examiners who know the individual to provide references, to provide comments about the individual as to the qualities the board considers to be necessary ingredients to be a good examiner. Not all nominations are accepted. Accepted examiners begin with an apprenticeship as question authors for the written examination, an opportunity to see them in a different setting and see how they interact. A balance is sought of individuals from private practice as well as academic settings. There was a time when being a board examiner might have been a greater hardship for those in a private practice to devote an entire week to the exam. As I understand it, some academic settings are asking the associate examiners to use some of their vacation time. If new examiners in the year of examinations seem to demonstrate a good likelihood of success as an associate examiner, they will be appointed to a two-year provisional appointment and invited to examine on two separate occasions. If they continue to show the ability to conduct good examinations and to grade appropriately, they will be appointed to a four-year term as an associate examiner, those terms are renewable. The board has not set a finite number of terms that an individual can serve as an associate examiner. The directors of the board must have been active associate examiners to be considered for election to directorship, so there is a progression there as well.

Dr. Albert B. Gerbie (American Board of Obstetrics and Gynecology): I'm the only one who has been in private practice for 43 years and never had a residency. The board has a rotation system of two years as associate and then five years as examiner. The examiners may take a furlough and return. The board tries to select residency program directors from non-university hospitals as examiners. On the other hand, it is very important, from the standpoint of the candidate, that examiners are practiced at evaluation; people who have been teaching and evaluating throughout their life are better prepared to evaluate a person and to understand some of the statistical problems in an evaluation.

Dr. Jose Biller (American Board of Psychiatry & Neurology): The oral exam is to some degree artificial and contrived to try to get through a lot of information quickly. Certainly, the candidates are concerned about being familiar with the format of the exam, the ground rules, gamesmanship, interactions. They prepare for these oral exams a little differently than their standard education in a residency, preparation often includes taking specific review courses to learn the gamesmanship involved and become familiar with the exam mechanics. My question is, to what degree are these exams measuring gamesmanship and specific preparation for these activities, as opposed to measuring the kind of clinical judgment and performance that I think the board really wants to measure?

Dr. Guerin: We would hope the exam is not measuring gamesmanship. We try to make ours clinically relevant and base it on, as has been said, whether they know the words and don't miss the tune, but we would hope they can all sing in harmony. We do not think there is much gaming. If it is identified, it might even be held against a candidate. I have not seen measuring gamesmanship as a problem in the board process.

Dr. Gerbie: Remember you can play games with the written exam. The board is very careful about going over the distractors in the written exam to be sure they are true distractors and not easily rejected, so a good test taker cannot play the exam in the written.

Dr. Mancall: Dr. Lunz, do you have a final comment on this question of gamesmanship and level playing fields?

Dr. Lunz: That is a pretty broad question, actually. From my perspective I guess I would say that, with any human interaction, you know there has to be a certain amount of gamesmanship. I seriously doubt that anyone here intends to measure that or that it is a primary factor in the examination process. One of the certifying boards I work with did an assessment of their oral protocols a few years ago. What they found was that the easy oral protocols were similar to "zero distractors" in multiple choice items: The protocol had one answer and candidates either knew it or didn't. Boards should be willing to look at some of the statistical ways to "level the playing field." These involve accounting for however the exam is intended to measure the content; not necessarily saying whether the intended assessment is good, bad or neutral, but just accounting for what happens in the examination process so that everybody has an equal opportunity to pass, if they're competent.

Dr. Scheiber: Just a final comment, I think a lot of candidates are very anxious. The best preparation for taking the exam is being a good resident in a good residency. Most people do not need expensive review courses to get through the exam process. Board review is a very expensive industry, candidates are spending a lot for an exercise that I think is unnecessary. Many of the things they learn their parents should have taught them when they were young. Things like "get a good night's sleep," "get washed in the morning," "wear a tie," "look like a doctor." I think they ought to go back to their parents for advice rather than spend a thousand dollars at a course!

PART 5

FROM ADAPTIVE TESTING TO AUTOMATED SCORING OF ARCHITECTURAL SIMULATIONS

From Adaptive Testing to Automated Scoring of Architectural Simulations

Isaac I. Bejar, Ph.D.
Educational Testing Service

In addressing the question of assessing professional reasoning and judgment it was helpful to review the accomplishments in medicine and health care and compare those efforts to the one's I am most familiar with in testing and measurement in general, and in other professions. A recent article that reviewed the past two decades of work in testing professional performance in the health professions provides a similar message to mine: "Use of a battery of [assessment] methods, combining efficient sampling of these clinically oriented written tests with complementary in-depth performance-based assessment of clinical skills, should be more successful than use of either family of methods in isolation, both psychometrically and educationally."[1]

Interestingly, these lessons in health care have been learned and applied in other professions with much success. My presentation will report on one of these efforts, the project to revise the licensure examination for architects: National Council of Architectural Registration Boards/Educational Testing Service Project (NCARB/ETS Project). The project aims to convert a paper-and-pencil examination to a fully computer-administered and computer-automated scoring of the examination with an implementation target date of 1997. The current examination consists of several multiple-choice formatted tests, and two "graphic" or open-ended questions which cover Building Design and Site Design. The revised examination will be administered only on computer and will comprise most of the current multiple-choice sections but administered in a computer-adaptive testing format; the two graphic sections will be replaced by corresponding open-ended computer-based simulations. In reporting our experience in this research and development project for licensing architects I hope you will appreciate four points:

1. An examination for assessing professionals for licensure or certification must meet at least these conditions: include multiple assessment methods which assess a variety of skills and knowledge, fit into a limited testing time period, and can strike a defensible and sensible balance between psychometric and economic considerations.
2. Computer-based testing offers a way to reduce the amount of testing time for using multiple-choice questions (computer-adaptive testing) to free up time for assessing open-ended performance.
3. Computer-based simulations which realistically simulate problems in architectural planning and design, can be developed economically after a learning period involving a multidisciplinary team.
4. Scoring of computer-based simulations can be done by computer algorithms that do not require further hand scoring by experts, except as a quality control procedure.

In describing how the project considered each of these points I hope to offer insights into the reasoning process we used to attain our goal of a totally computer-based examination including scoring the simulations.

The Design Strategy Used in the NCARB/ETS Project

The examination design problem for the NCARB/ETS Project has a number of threads which lead to creating a totally computer-based multiple-method examination. On the one hand, the psychometric community has debated for many years the issue of the superiority of closed-ended questions (multiple-choice questions) versus open-ended questions (essay questions). The tension created by these debates leads naturally to the conclusion that a combination of different question formats resulting in different response modalities from examinees may be the ideal approach to measure a complex skill.[2] The project adopted the strategy of integrating both questioning formats on a computer-based examination platform.

An issue faced by the project was the recognition that performance-based assessments using open-ended questions take more testing time than closed-ended questions per unit of information gathered from examinees. In computer assessments testing time is expensive, but the time spent by examinees on the computer can be quantified precisely and conveniently. Also, administering examinations on computers allows greater flexibility in allocation of time spent on various test modalities.

One way of reducing the testing time for multiple-choice questions is to use *computer adaptive testing (CAT)*. In CAT each examinee receives the minimum number of test questions until a decision can be reached about the examinee's ability (classify them as passing or failing). Frequently for examinees who are poorly prepared or superbly prepared, a test using multiple-choice questions can be reduced considerably with CAT compared to the equivalent paper-and-pencil version, provided an adequate item pool exists. The time saved by using CAT can then be devoted to assessing open-ended performance. The CAT format maintains the test reliability even with fewer items, saves time in test administration, but requires a much larger test item pool than conventional paper-and-pencil tests, and the test items must be carefully calibrated and coded for difficulty and content.[3]

Although much research had been done on CAT, by the 1980s none of the existing procedures were totally suited to the NCARB exam. Therefore, the first phase of the research and development program was to develop an operational computer-adaptive testing system for use in licensing decisions. The system was developed and field tested successfully in 1988. Based on that successful field test, it was possible to estimate the savings in testing time that would be possible through adaptive testing. That information became part of the knowledge base needed to design the more complex transition from paper-and-pencil graphic exams to the fully computer-administered and computer-scored performance aspects of the exam. Although the approach was motivated by an examination designed for architects, it is completely general and has been applied in other professions.[4] Details of the approach can be found in Lewis and Sheehan.[5]

Computer-Based Simulations

The second phase of the project was devoted to the development of the simulation segment of the licensure examination. There were two major tasks: Conceptualization and implementation of a pool of test items (i.e.,computer-based simulations or vignettes); and design and implementation procedures leading to automated scoring of performance on the simulations. The building of an item pool of vignettes was informed by a *job analysis*. The job analysis procedure in professional assessment enumerates and rates the importance of skills expected of an individual in the defined professional role (American Psychological Association Standards).[6] Using an iterative procedure the job analysis data provides both the context of the vignettes and the specific tasks expected to be performed in the simulation. Each vignette type was developed in sufficient detail so that a committee of expert architects could define a small number of solutions. The solutions served as the basis for formulating the scoring rules.

This process required a multidisciplinary team consisting of computer scientists, architects and measurement experts. Although it was a laborious task and a major undertaking, the resulting library of simulations classified by the tasks being measured provided clear advantages. Thinking of problem classes rather than of specific problems forced the test developers to spell out in detail the specifications of each problem class. Creating additional vignettes for a problem class, however, became less difficult knowing the intended measurement goal for the problem class.

Among the specifications defining a problem class are:

- **Program statement**. The program statement is the problem as presented to the candidate. The specifications cover both linguistic and graphic considerations. Linguistic ambiguities are removed through tight control over the language used to express program statements. Similarly, controlling the graphic characteristics makes it possible to control the difficulty of different instances of the problem class. Further control of difficulty among instances is obtained by setting guidelines for maintaining equivalence of key design constraints.
- **Scoring tree**. The scoring tree refers to the aspects of a solution that will be taken into account as part of scoring. The scoring tree and the program statement are strongly linked because the scoring tree contains weights for different kinds of errors, for example. Therefore, the chance of committing errors must be held approximately constant across different instances of the problem class.
- **Interface**. The interface provided for a given problem type must be applicable with equal ease to all instances of that problem type. As with every component of the system, the process of interface development is iterative and uses field trials to obtain empirical data. A draft interface is developed using the committee's best judgment. It is then tried with candidates ranging in computing experience. Adjustments are made as necessary for a given problem type while keeping in mind the interface for all the other problem classes. The goal throughout the process is to streamline the interface while keeping it as consistent as possible across vignettes in a problem class and between problem classes.

It is fair to say that this approach to task development is resource intensive, at least initially. The expectation is that the payoff will occur in the form of savings when we create more vignettes for a problem class, as well as defining entirely new classes. A significant amount of learning has taken place in the development process and this learning can be leveraged to expand the assessment to other skills.

The Scoring Approach

The approach to test design outlined in the previous section was, in part, motivated by the need to develop automated scoring procedures that would be applicable to multiple problems. Early research on scoring focused on demonstrations of feasibility with single problems. This early research demonstrated that, by suitably representing solutions to design problems, it was possible to emulate the judgments that human graders made about the problems.[7,8] Although the results were reassuring and much was learned from them, they did not address the question of applying the scoring procedure across vignettes in the problem class. An important advantage of automated scoring is the capability of scoring, unassisted, all instances of a given problem class (i.e., the scoring procedure is across vignettes and across problem classes). Clearly, the next challenge was to collect data on several vignettes designed to be equivalent and from the same problem class. The first opportunity to thoroughly test this scoring procedure will be during the national field test to be carried out in 1996.

The scoring method relies on a knowledge elicitation and representation approach developed by Henry Braun. The method produces a treelike or hierarchical organization of problem features needed to characterize performance on a problem class or vignette type. This scoring method has several advantages but its main value is that architects have accepted it and are comfortable with it.

As an illustration consider the design problem of planning a bathroom displayed in Figure 1.

Figure 1. Bathroom Design Problem

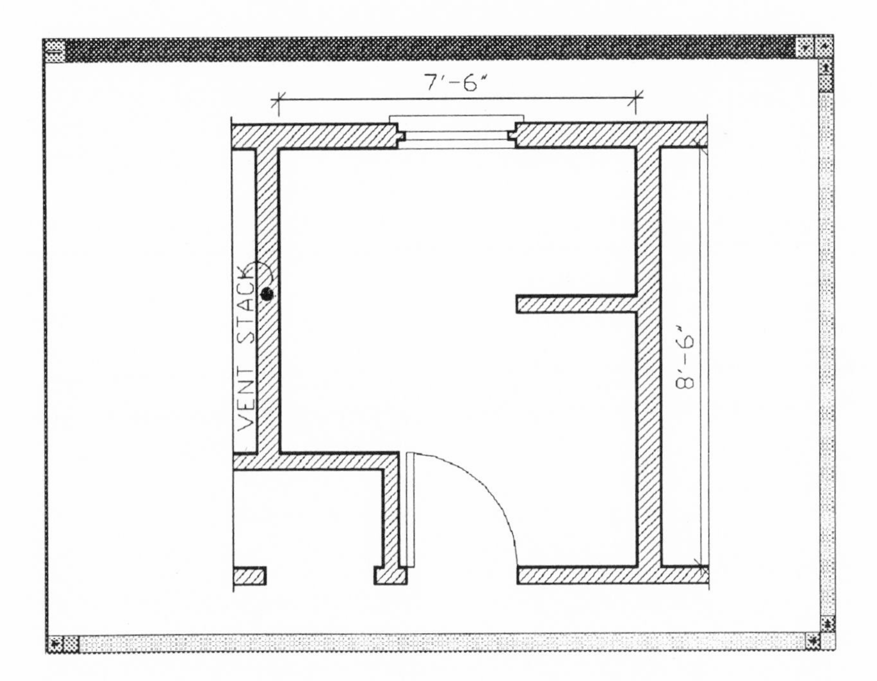

This is what the candidate would see on the computer screen with the icons on the left serving as the interface for the candidate to enter and solve the problem. By pressing the *space bar* on the computer keyboard the candidate can refer to the problem to be resolved as well as access relevant reference material. Clicking on the *Draw icon* offers the candidate a menu of design objects that can be placed in the solution, such as a bathtub, toilet, etc. The other icons allow the candidate a series of actions to refine the solution, such as moving and rotating the different design elements.

Good and not so good solutions to this bathroom design problem are displayed in Figures 2 and 3.

Figure 2 Bathroom Design Solution #1

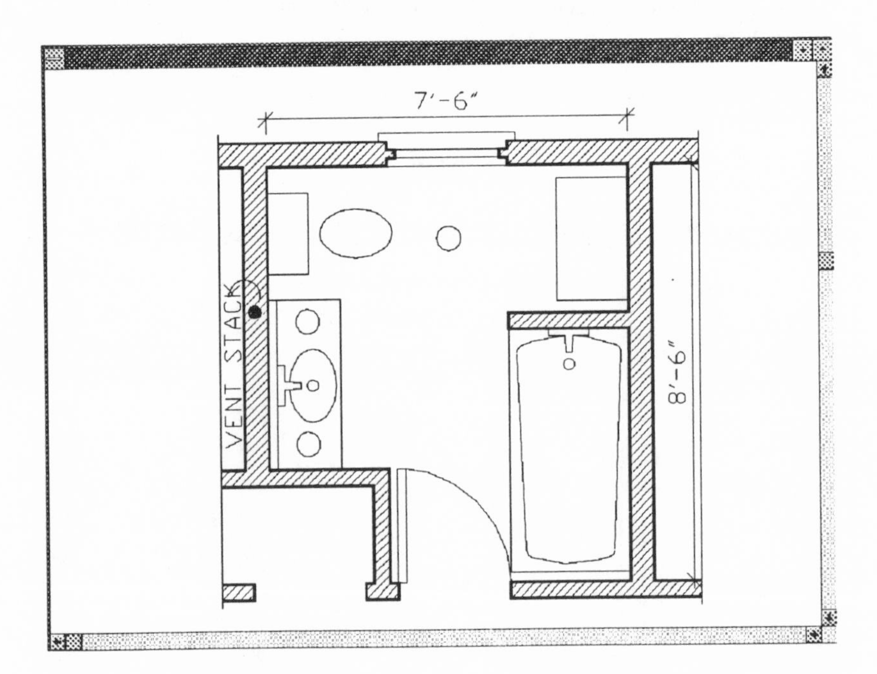

Figure 3. Bathroom Design Solution #2

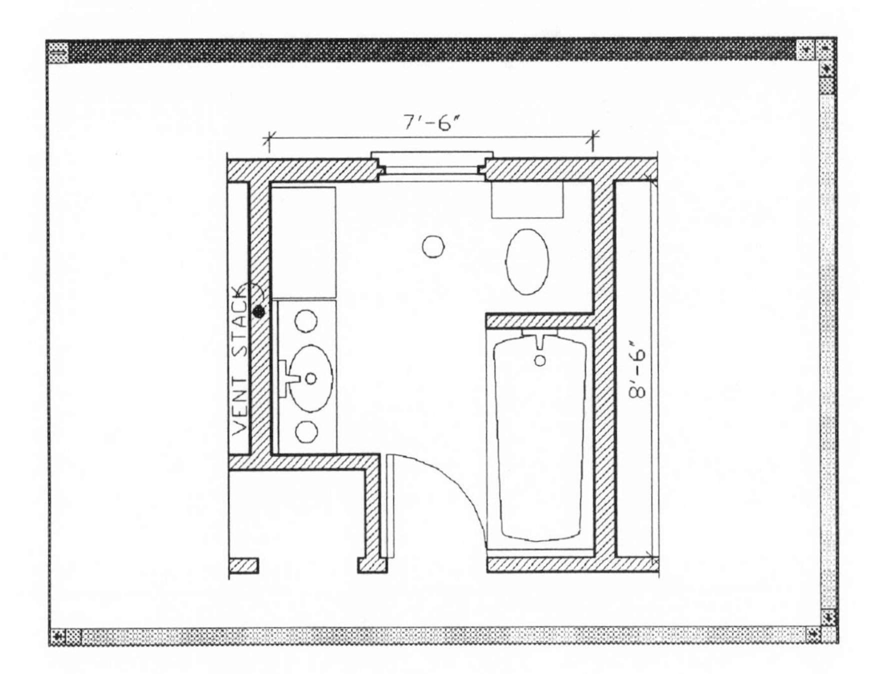

A scoring tree for this problem can be seen in Figure 4.

Figure 4. Bathroom Remodel Evaluation Map

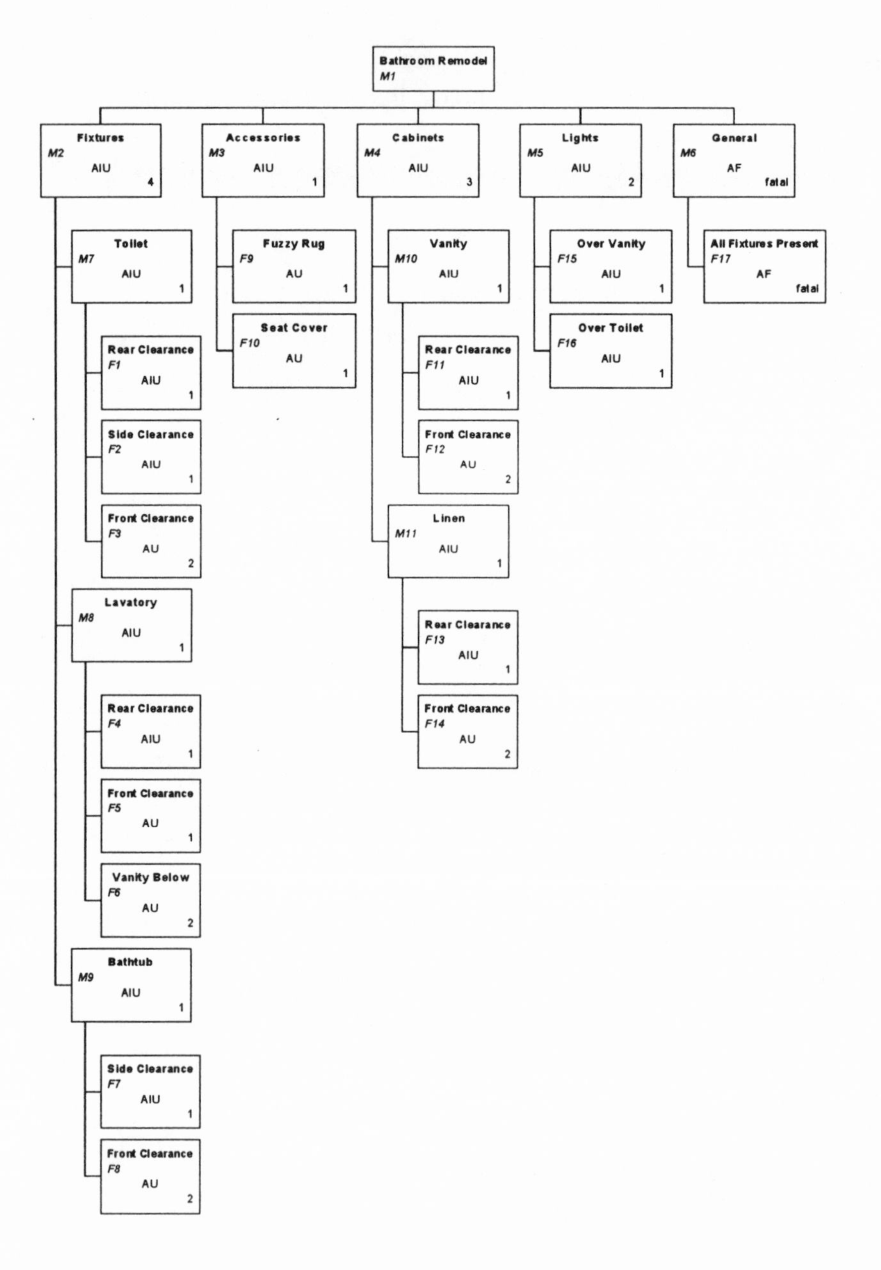

Scoring trees are formulated initially as a top-down process where the architects, based on their experience grading open-ended problems in the paper-and-pencil test, formulate broad categories that characterize the solution to a type of problem. The broad categories, for example, design logic, are not directly computable from the representation of a solution and, therefore, need to be fleshed out into more basic characterizations that are, in fact, computable. The process is arduous and it involves, in addition to architects, computer scientists and test developers. We have found that a hierarchical tree representation is both a natural and convenient form of knowledge elicitation.[9]

There are basically two types of nodes in the scoring tree hierarchy. One type consists of low-level features requiring a direct computation from the solution, such as computing the location of an element, the distance between design elements, or counting the presence or absence of some elements. The outcome of each feature is a classification into one of three categories: Acceptable (A), Indeterminate (I), and Unacceptable (U). Initially the thresholds for the categories are set judgmentally, based on the collective expertise of the architects involved in the project. As data is collected, however, the thresholds are revisited and adjusted as necessary.

The second type of node consists of clusters of lower-level features. Again, the lower level or clusters are subsumed under a given higher cluster which is already completed. Indeed, the computation of a vignette score proceeds from the computation of the lower-level features upward in the order dictated by the tree.

Features and clusters scores take three values: A, I, or U. In the case of the Fixtures cluster (See Figure 4), which is composed of three lower-level features, there are 27 (3x3x3) different possible "input" feature values; these are partially enumerated in Table 1. Each such outcome can be summarized by the counts of any two of the three possible values. We have used the U's and I's as the summary of an outcome measure as seen in the last two columns of Table 1. All possible values for a cluster can be represented by a two-dimensional matrix where the rows refer to the number of I's and the columns refer to the number of U's.

Table 1. Enumeration of Feature Values Corresponding to Toilet, Lavatory and Bathtub Clusters

Feature Value Sets	Fixture Cluster			Counts	
	Toilet	Lavatory	Bathtub	U	I
1.	A	A	A	0	0
2.	I	A	A	0	1
3.	A	I	A	0	1
4.	A	A	I	0	1
5.	I	I	A	0	2
6.	I	A	I	0	2
7.	A	I	I	0	2
8.	I	I	I	0	3
9.	U	A	A	1	0
10.	A	U	A	1	0
11.	I	U	I	2	2
12.	U	I	I	1	2
.	.	.	.	.	.
.	.	.	.	.	.
27.	U	U	U	3	0

Note: U = Unacceptable I = Indeterminate A = acceptable

Table 2 is a possible matrix for the Fixture cluster. According to this matrix, an "A" corresponds to feature value set #1 with zero I's and Zero U's (e.g., the feature value set #1 in Table 1). An "I" corresponds to feature value set number with one I and zero U's (e.g., feature value sets #2, #3, and #4 in Table 1.) All other feature value sets get assigned a U.

Table 2. Summary Matrix for Fixture Cluster

		U's		
		0	1	2
I's	0	A	U	U
	1	I	U	U
	2	U	U	U
	3	U	U	U

The matrix approach to summarize scores has been found to be a convenient format to rank the feature cluster measures, and locate two cut scores to identify the combinations associated with an A, I or U score. The initial process is modified each time there are changes in problem specifications or other information. Data collected from field trials are used to suggest further changes. For example, some features may be found not to function well, or be ambiguously defined, or computationally infeasible as originally conceived. Any potential changes are considered very cautiously because all the other instances of the vignette type must be considered in order to avoid the introduction of instance-specific scoring considerations. Occasionally, from such considerations emerges a need to revise the specifications. For example, the initial specifications for the vignette type concerned with lighting and ventilation allowed for the possibility of one or two air supplies and returns. After data was collected on this vignette type, this flexibility was found to be problematic and eliminated.

Conclusions

The NCARB/ETS project is based on the idea that thoughtful application of computers to assessment can lead to significant improvements in scoring decisions, not just examination efficiency. Computer adaptive testing (CAT) is one such thoughtful application and plays a significant role in improving the quality of decisions based on test scores. Through computer-adaptive testing it is possible to improve the precision of scores using multiple-choice questions as well as reduce testing time. The savings in time can then be devoted to assess performance by means of open-ended, high-fidelity formats such as computer-based simulations.

Having the flexibility to devote more time to open-ended formats is one mechanism for dealing with the task specificity problem which has plagued simulation-based assessment. The additional testing time made possible by the use of adaptive testing must be used well, however, to ensure that as much ground is being covered in the allocated time for assessing open-ended performance. For example, the computer interface must be powerful and easily learnable, and yet consistent across different types of vignettes. Efficient interfaces will not suffice, however. The key to the task specificity problem may lie in a deeper understanding of the nature of professional expertise and the careful design of tasks to elicit that expertise in an examination context. We have outlined above some of the specific steps we have taken to minimize construct-irrelevant variance and to control the difficulty of problems through a deeper understanding of the architectural design process. That deeper understanding comes from cognitive analyses of performances and tasks[10,11] as well as from the multidisciplinary discussions involved in the process of computerizing the delivery and scoring of problems.[9]

Acknowledgments

I am greatly indebted to Philip Bashook for helping to clarify the points in this paper. I am also grateful to Henry Braun and Brent Bridgeman for reviews of earlier drafts that were also helpful.

References

1. Swanson DB, Norman GR, Linn RL. Performance-Based Assessment Lessons from the Health Professions, *Educ Res* 1995; 24:5-11, 35.

2. Ackerman PL, Smith TA. A comparison of the information provided by essay, multiple-choice and free-response writing tests. *Appl Psychol Measure* 1988;12:117-128.

3. Wainer H, Dorans NJ, Green BF, Flaugher R, Mislevy RJ, Steinberg L, Thissen D. *Computerized adaptive testing: A primer*. Hillsdale, NJ: Lawrence Erlbaum Associates; 1990.

4. Lewis C, Smith RL. *Using a new computerized mastery testing model.* Paper presented at the annual meeting of the National Council on Measurement in Education, San Francisco, CA, 1990.

5. Lewis C, Sheehan K. Using Beyesian decision theory to design a computerized mastery test. *App Psychol Measure* 1990;14(4):367-386.

6. American Educational Research Association (AERA); American Psychological Association (APA); National Council on Measurement in Education (NCME); Joint Committee (1985); *Standards for Educational and Psychological Testing, Revised 1985.* Washington, DC: American Psychological Association, 1985.

7. Bejar II. A methodology for scoring open-ended architectural design problems. *J Appl Psychol* 1991;76:522-532.

8. Oltman PK, Bejar II, Kim SH. *An approach to automated scoring of architectural designs.* Proceedings of Fifth International Conference on Computer-aided Architectural Design edited by Fleming U and Van Wik S., July 1993, New York, New York (pp. 215-224).

9. Bejar II, Braun HI. On the synergy between assessment and instruction: Early lessons from computer-based simulations. *Machine-Mediated Learning*, 1994;4(1):5-25.

10. Akin O. *Calibration of Problem Difficulty: In Architectural Design Problems Designed for the Automated Licensing Examination System in the United States of America.* Unpublished manuscript, 1994.

11. Katz IR. *From laboratory to test booklet: Using expert-novice comparisons to guide design of performance assessment* (Unpublished manuscript ed.). Princeton: Educational Testing Services, 1994.

ALTERNATIVES TO THE STANDARDIZED ORAL EXAMINATION

PART 6

The Key Feature Examination: a Written Test of Decision-Making Skills

W. Dale Dauphinee, M.D., FRCPC
The Medical Council of Canada

In the summer of 1984, a group of international and local experts in medical education met at the First Cambridge Conference on Medical Education to discuss the current state of clinical assessment. The conference was designed to permit a frank exchange of ideas in a think-tank environment. One of the subgroups focused on recent innovations in the evaluation of clinical competence. Those innovations covered the spectrum from written examinations to standardized patients to computer simulations. In the published summary and review of the literature arising from the subgroup's discussion, Norman made the following comment.

> "In many cases, considerable research evidence has accrued to indicate that these new methods have value as assessment and learning devices. Conversely, research on many of the traditional measures of competence, such as global summative rating scales, essay tests and multiple-choice examinations has shown severe deficiencies in reliability, validity or both. Yes, despite these research findings, assessment by medical schools and licensing bodies is dominated by these methods, and other innovations have had relatively little impact."[1]

In addition to reviewing the field, Norman and collaborators made a number of suggestions for a future research agenda, including the assessment of problem-solving or clinical reasoning. It was noted that "clinical problem-solving isunlikely to represent a general skill, but rather is a reflection of the application and synthesis of knowledge to the solution of specific problems."[1] The group proposed that "Cambridge Cases" be developed which would represent a unique clinical challenge and that the solution to the clinical problem of each case would focus on a few "essential elements of the problem."

Two other developments at that time also contributed to the medical educators' perception of the need for a shift in the assessment of clinical reasoning. One was the realization that the current approach, using patient management problems (PMPs) was flawed.[2,3] In 1983 Norcini, Swanson and Webster found that multiple-choice questions (MCQs) were more reliable and efficient in the use of testing time than PMPs, and that PMPs assessed the same components of clinical competence as did the MCQ format.[2] In a second study in 1984, Norcini, Swanson, Grosso, and Webster looked at alternative methods for scoring PMPs which might improve their measurement qualities and found that none of the alternative scoring systems improved the performance of the PMPs.[3] The issue was well summarized in Bordage and Page's first publication about the "key features" concept, an alternative approach to patient management problems.[4] As Norman once commented, PMPs took too long to do too little.[5] A decade or so earlier, LaDuca at Hahnemann and his colleagues developed the notion of the Professional Performance Situation Model.[6] This model defined physician expertise in terms of the relationship between performance tasks and professional context. This concept of the situational perspective led to the crossing of conventional disciplinary boundaries and focusing on the physician's intervention in FLEX II (Federation Licensing Examination).[7]

The second major influence was the progress in understanding of clinical decision-making skills. This was summarized in Norman's analysis of the research on the nature of clinical decision making from the first Cambridge Conference.[1] The essential point was that problem-solving skills were specific to the case or problem presented and that those skills required the effective manipulation of a few essential elements which were critical to the successful resolution of the problem. Page and Bordage later used the expression "key features" and pointed out that: "Key features are unique for each problem."[8]

As a result of the first Cambridge Conference, some of the attendees from Canada pursued the idea of developing a new test to replace the PMPs which constituted one of the four written papers of the Qualifying Examination of The Medical Council of Canada (MCC). The MCC has the responsibility for providing a national examination acceptable as the basis for licensure for all provincial medical licensing authorities in Canada. The MCC approved the project in 1986 and, after development, the "key features approach" officially replaced the PMPs in 1992 as one of the four components or question books in the MCC's Qualifying Examination taken at the end of medical curriculum. It was known as the Q4 project because it was the fourth question booklet of the two-day examination! Essentially, a key features examination is composed of many short cases, each focusing on essential or critical aspects of the identification andmanagement of the case, i.e., the key features. The development of the project is the subject of a series of four articles recently appearing in *Academic Medi-*

cine under the authorship of the two principal investigators, Dr. Georges Bordage and Dr. Gordon Page and their co-workers.[8,9,10,11]

The purpose of this presentation is to review the key feature component of the MCC Qualifying Examination Part I from three perspectives: 1) a description of the structure of the examination; 2) a brief review of the validation studies of the key features; and 3) its current status. The technical features of its development are covered in the *Academic Medicine* series and will not be commented on here.

The Structure of the Test

The current Medical Council of Canada Qualifying Examination has two parts. Part I is a two-day written examination taken at the end of the medical undergraduate program and consists of four one-half-day components. The first three components use MCQs consisting of 520 written and pictorial items with clinical stems. The fourth component is the key feature test of clinical decision making. It makes up one-quarter of the total score for Part I. It is the subject of this presentation. Part II is a 20-station Objective Structured Clinical Examination utilizing standardized patients lasting one-half-day and taken after 15 months of postgraduate clinical training.[12] Both Parts I and II must be passed to achieve the Licentiate of The Medical Council of Canada. All examinations are criterion-referenced.

The key feature portion of Part I consists of a booklet of about 32 clinical cases which in turn generate a total of about 70 questions focusing on a critical element or key features; (i.e., two or three key features per case). The key features test thereby permits a greater sampling of the domain and consequently improves the reliability as compared to the old test of PMPs which typically contained 12 to 15 problems. The key feature approach also permits a flexible approach to test item format, minimizes the opportunity for cuing, and can accommodate more complex sets of responses that may be required to resolve the problem.

Several steps are involved in the development of the key feature cases and examination. The published discipline-based objectives of the MCC define the domain to be tested.[13] Within these objectives, each problem is stated in terms of a presenting complaint (e.g., upper gastrointestinal hemorrhage). The presenting complaints in toto, as defined in the objectives, constitute the domain for testing in the key feature portion of the examination. The blueprint for the key features portion of the examination is based on the human life span broken into five periods: pregnancy, neonatal and infant (up to one year), pediatrics (1-11 years), adolescence (12-18), adulthood, and geriatrics (65 and older). The relative proportion of each of the life periods depicted on the examination is based on representative figures of the distribution of medical services for Canadians in each age group.

Each case must outline a clinical situation for the problem. The key features must be defined in advance before that case is developed. Thus the key features for each clinical situation are discussed, refined and agreed upon by the test committee before each test case is written. The term clinical situation refers to the way in which the patient would present with the problem to the physician. Any one or more of the five following situations can be defined for each problem:

1. An undifferentiated complaint or problem.
2. A single typical case.
3. A multiple or multi-system problem.
4. A life-threatening situation.
5. A preventive care or health promotion situation.

A typical problem would have two to three key features, but as few as one and as many as five have been used. An example may help:

Figure 1. Example of Key Features Clinical Interaction (Skeleton)

An adult presents complaining of a painful, swollen leg.

The physician should demonstrate the following key features to resolve the problem:

Key Features:

1. Include deep vein thrombosis in the differential diagnosis.
2. Elicit the risk factors for deep vein thrombosis from the patient's history.
3. Order a venogram as the definitive test for deep vein thrombosis.

The case scenario is then developed around this skeleton. Once the case is developed, each question typically focuses on one key feature. If cuing could arise from testing more than one key feature per problem, another case can be used to test the other key feature. The third key feature of the painful leg example, ordering a venogram, illustrates that problem. Therefore, a separate case is developed to test that feature.

Two formats of questions are used; short answer write-ins and short menu multiple-choice. As one might suspect, in the write-in questions candidates supply their own answers by simply writing in the response on the answer sheet. In the case of short menu questions, the candidate selects the response from a given list of options. The number of options vary but are usually between 15 to

20 and infrequently have been over 40. In order to avoid cuing or guessing, anticipated misconceptions or plain wrong responses, attractive responses are included on the menus to serve as good distractors. At one time a long menu (i.e., in a booklet) was considered but was discarded as impractical. Generally, write-in questions are reserved for situations eliciting diagnosis and treatment decisions.

The scoring key consists of the list of correct responses. Some scoring keys have only one correct response and others may have several. To illustrate, in the example of the patient with a painful, swollen leg, there were at least five items from the list of eight on the history which must be identified to obtain a score of "1." The scoring is dichotomous, that is either "0" or "1." The option of assigning partial scores of up to "1" can be used, for example 2/5, etc., but the maximum per question is still "1." Some scoring keys require a score of "0" for a particular action, no matter what else the candidate chooses because the action may be dangerous or harmful. The test score becomes the sum of individual problem scores; problems are equally weighted regardless of the number of key features per problem. *The unit of measurement is the case, not the key feature.*

Like all of The Medical Council of Canada's examinations, the key feature test is criterion-referenced. The test committee, along with the other discipline committees and the Central Examination Committee, sets passing level standards using the Angoff method, before final approval is given for the test to be used in Part I.

Examples of key feature cases and the scoring keys are presented in the information pamphlet for the Medical Council of Canada Qualifying Examination Part I.[14]

Validation of Key Features

Page and Bordage, in their development work, conducted a two-part study to validate the key features methodology for the Part I examination.[10] The purpose of the studies was to establish the content validity of the key features method. A target group of 99 physicians directly involved in clerkship programs at the 16 Canadian schools were asked to estimate clinical clerks' frequency of exposure to the problems in the key features test item bank. One study was done retrospectively judging existing key features and one was prospective generating key features. The retrospective study showed that 92 percent of the key features were corroborated by the outside physicians and 94 percent were corroborated in the prospective study. Of the problems in the bank, 37 percent were estimated to have been seen once in the clerkship, 46 percent to have been seen three to five times, and 17 percent to have been seen six times or more. Thus, Bordage and colleagues concluded that the committee's definition of key features is very similar to medical school faculty members' perspective and that the key-feature problems are generally representative of clinical situations seen by senior students during clinical clerkships in Canada.

The Current Experience and Results

The newly developed test was field tested with small groups of volunteers first, then by pilot testing in the 1991 MCC examinations; it was introduced in 1992 into Part I. Since 1992, it has been used as one of the four booklets of Part I. The experience to date has been very positive. The test has not presented any logistic problems. There have been discussions about how much time candidates should have for this test (3 and 1/2 hours or 4 hours?). Currently, it is four hours in duration, averaging 70 actual cases. There are twelve pilot cases introduced each year (12 new cases times five parallel examination formats for a total of 60 new cases).

What has been the qualitative assessment of the test? First, it is easy to administer. From that point of view, on entering the examination site, if one did not look over the students' shoulders and watch their workbooks, it would look like another written MCQ formatted examination. Second, the students enjoy the examination. One does not hear complaints that the test is assessing only recall and being a test of memory. Students know that completeness and compulsiveness are not rewarded. Third, a major difference is the marking of the "write-in items." This requires knowledgeable individuals to read the write-ins and assess the answer against the possible acceptable answers; there was shown to be an 18 percent difference in scores between write-ins and short menus, write-ins being harder. There can be more than one acceptable answer. Synonyms have to be evaluated. This is typically done over a weekend by 12 postgraduate trainees who have passed the examination previously (accompanied by lots of pizza!). If there is doubt about a write-in, the test committee secretary and chair make a final decision. The corrected responses are scored and data transferred to scoring sheets. Along with the short-menu responses, all are entered into a computer by optical scanner for further statistical analyses.

What has been the reliability data on the key features format in Part I? Table 1 summarizes the reliability data using Cronbach's alpha for the Q4 component and all components of the Part I examination for the years 1992 to 1994. The exam has not yet been given in 1995.

Table 1. Reliability Estimates For the Q4 and the Total MCCQE Part I by Year (Cronbach's Alpha)

Examination Component	1992	1993	1994
Q4 Only	0.75	0.74	0.72
All Components	0.91	0.92	0.91

The final Part I score is based on four booklets; three are made up of MCQ questions and the fourth is the key features question. The overall test has performed well. Nonetheless, the goal is to increase the reliability for the fourth question set (key features).

Concerns about the reliability and question quality of the key feature examination will be addressed in a major workshop this year. Some of the issues will be: Increasing the number of problems but leaving the time at four hours; focusing on problems and not questions in the blueprint; refocusing the committee on improving and updating the current test item bank and slowing down the production of new problems.

Conclusions

The MCC are pleased with the first three years of experience with the key features examination. It is easy to administer. It covers more content areas in the same testing time as PMPs. It is congruent with current research findings about medical decision making. There is less cuing. It does not reward completeness unless required, nor shotgun approaches. Students like it. Residents can mark the write-in questions and seem to enjoy it. Finally, the validity of the key-feature approach has been documented. The next challenge will be to adapt the approach to computer-based formats, to conduct studies of concurrent validity against other evaluation methods, and to carry out predictive validity studies in the context of proposed physician-monitoring programs using other data bases.

Acknowledgements

The author and The Medical Council of Canada wish to recognize the major contributions of Drs. Georges Bordage and Gordon Page, the principal investigators; Dr. Ian Bowmer, project coordinator; the members of the Q4 Test Committee; Dr. Louis Lavesseur, former Chair of the Central Examination Committee; and Dr. Michel Berard, Registrar Emeritus, in bringing the key features project from an idea to reality.

References

1. Norman G, Bordage G, Curry L, Dauphinee D. A review of recent innovations in assessment. In: *Directions in Clinical Assessment: Report of the First Cambridge Conference on the Assessment of Clinical Competence,* R. Wakeford, etc., Addenbrooke's Hospital, Cambridge: Cambridge University School of Clinical Medicine; 1985 pp. 8-27.

2. Norcini JJ, Swanson DB, Webster GD. Reliability, validity, and efficiency of various item formats in the assessment of physicians. *Proceedings* of Ann Conf Res Med Educ Assoc Am Med Coll; 1983 pp. 53-58.

3. Norcini JJ, Swanson DB, Grosso LJ, Webster GD. A comparison of several methods for scoring patient management problems. *Proceedings* of Ann Conf Res Med Educ Assoc Am Med Coll; 1984; pp. 41-46.

4. Bordage G, Page G. An alternative approach to PMPs: the "key features" concept. In I. Hart and R. Harden, (Eds.): *Further Developments in Assessing Clinical Competence,* Montreal: Can-Heal Publications; 1987 pp. 57-75.

5. Norman G. Striking the balance. *Acad Med* 1994; 69:209-210.

6. LaDuca A. The structure of competence in health professions. *Eval & Hlth Prof* 1980; 3:253-288.

7. LaDuca A, Taylor DD, Hill IK. The design of a new physician licensure examination. *Eval & Hlth Prof* 1984; 7:115-140.

8. Page G, Bordage G. A more valid written examination of clinical decision-making skills: The Medical Council of Canada's key feature project. *Acad Med 1995 70:104-110.*

9. Page G, Bordage G, Allen T. Developing key feature problems and examinations to assess clinical decision-making skills. *Acad Med* 1995 70:194-201.

10. Bordage G, Brailovsky C, Carretier H, Page G. Content validation of key features on a national examination of clinical decision-making skills. *Acad Med* 1995 70:276-281.

11. Bordage G, Carretier H, Bertrand R, Page G. Comparing time and performance of French- and English-speaking candidates taking a national examination of clinical decision-making skills. *Acad Med* 1995; 70:359-365.

12. Resnick RK, Blackmore DE, Cohen R, Baumber J et al. An Objective Structured Clinical Examination for the licentiate of The Medical Council of Canada: from research to reality. *Acad Med* 1993; 68:S4-S6.

13. Baumber J (Ed.). *Objectives of the Medical Council of Canada Qualifying Examination.* Ottawa: The Medical Council of Canada; 1992.

14. *Information Pamphlet on The Qualifying Examination Part I.* Ottawa: The Medical Council of Canada; 1995.

Computer-Based Case Simulations

Stephen G. Clyman, M.D.
Donald E. Melnick, M.D.
Brian E. Clauser, Ed.D.
National Board of Medical Examiners

What is CBX?

CBX is a computer program that simulates a patient/physician encounter by presenting an examinee with an unknown clinical problem allowing the examinee to care for the patient's unfolding situation. The computer records each step in the care of the patient and scores the performance of the doctor. The physician obtains information by requesting a history and/or physical examination, ordering laboratory studies, procedures, and consultants. He or she must balance the clinical information available with evidence of the acuity of the clinical problem in deciding what treatments to begin and when. Progression of the disease and the effects of treatments must be monitored, again using history, physical examination, and laboratory studies.

The computer simulates an environment familiar to all physicians. Orders for tests, treatments, hospitalization, etc., are written on an order sheet.The program will accept orders for thousands of different tests and treatments. A "clerk" verifies the accuracy of the orders. The patient can be seen in the office or the emergency department and/or admitted to the hospital, either to a ward or intensive care environment. The patient's chart contains the expected records; vital signs and medication records, notes describing history, physical examination, and procedures, nurses' notes, and results of tests.

A major feature of CBX is the simulation of time. The physician controls the movement of time. The clock moves forward (and the patient's condition changes) only when the physician initiates the movement of time. Although time cannot be reversed, the movement of time can be suspended while the doctor considers next steps. As a result, CBX records physician decision making over time in an unfolding clinical situation.

After the physician completes the care of a number of patients, the computer program compares the care strategies employed with those defined by expert panels and tested with many physicians. Physicians score higher when their actions are closer to those defined as ideal. This scoring system avoids rewarding thoroughness at the expense of efficiency. Risky, dangerous, or otherwise unindicated commissions and dangerous omissions in patient care are tracked and may have a substantial impact on the final scores.

Why is the CBX Format Useful?

CBX allows evaluation of patient care strategies. These strategies are captured in a realistic context, without artificial cues or segregation of the component tasks that make up patient management. For educational purposes, the care of patients is often segregated into individual tasks; differential diagnosis, laboratory studies, diagnosis, and treatment. However, this is a highly artificial representation of the actual sequence of events in caring for real patients. In real life, the diagnosis unfolds, often as a result of observed responses to treatment. Differential diagnoses change from hour to hour or day to day as the available clinical information changes. The diagnosis is not an endpoint; rather, it is a step in the total care of the patient. Effective monitoring of changes in the patient's condition because of the disease and/or its treatment is as important as accurate diagnosis in the outcome for the patient.

The totality of patient care is more than the simple sum of its constituent parts. The complex interplay of clinical information about the patient with time and physician action cannot be accurately and comprehensively represented and evaluated by the separation of patient care into many individual parts. Furthermore, testing methods that reduce care of a patient into a series of questions necessarily provide artificial cues that become unnatural and affect examinee responses. CBX is designed to avoid unnatural cuing by providing only those cues that would occur in the real world.

CBX is useful, therefore, because it allows the evaluation of important patient care skills in a more realistic and integrated manner than other available testing methods.

What Does CBX NOT Do?

CBX is designed to maximize information about physician decision-making while caring for specific patients. *It does not gather information regarding the adequacy of history-taking or physical examination skills.* In order to simplify the computer program and the scoring, and because it is less germane to the objective of CBX testing, doctors are not asked to specify doses or dosing frequency when ordering drugs. Currently the examinee is also not asked to make a diagnosis; but the new version of CBX, due for completion in 1995, will require entry of presumptive diagnoses at key points.

The patient in CBX responds to treatment as defined by the author of the case. CBX does not apply a probabilistic algorithm in deciding how the patient responds to a given intervention. This feature, while unlike the real world, assures that the stimulus presented is identical when examinees care for the patient in the same manner.

Because of the high cost and limited availability of image and sound delivery technology, CBX does not currently present visual images or sounds. Early versions of CBX successfully incorporated the presentation of images for common examination and laboratory test results. These features can be activated again in CBX when the test administration infrastructure makes it feasible. Use of a short video sequence is under investigation for display at the beginning of the case to convey the patient's overall condition, body habitus, comfort level, and other information.

How Does CBX Compare With Other Testing Methods?

CBX simulations complement simulations using standardized patients (SPs). "Standardized patients are people, with or without actual disease, who have been trained to portray a medical case in a consistent fashion."[1] Standardized patients gather information from a live patient about examinee interactions that are not represented easily in other formats. These include conversational (e.g., history taking, patient education, communication of bad news), behavioral (e.g., demeanor, professionalism, etc.), and psychomotor (e.g., physical examination) elements of the physician-patient interaction.

SP simulations do not assess effectively patient care over time, and they are relatively inefficient at gathering information regarding diagnosis and treatment. On the other hand, the SP method has the unique capacity to assess effectively history-taking, physical examination, and patient communication skills. CBX largely ignores the latter skills, but assesses patient care over time effectively.

Multiple-choice questions (MCQs) are highly efficient at assessing application of information in a constrained situation. They allow efficient sampling of broad domains of knowledge, producing highly stable measurements. No matter how clinically oriented they are, however, MCQs do not allow the presentation of dynamically unfolding clinical case presentations without artificially cuing the examinee. Studies comparing student performance on CBX and MCQs are described below. Of particular note is the finding that some students who do well on and would pass MCQ examinations do poorly on CBX examinations and likely would fail. The converse is also true. Thus, each method seems to provide unique information about the examinee and contributes to the pass/fail or mastery/non-mastery decision.

How is CBX Scored?

Scoring produces a measure of examinee performance by applying patient care criteria defined by experts to the actions taken by examinees on CBX cases. CBX scoring is expert based. Details of actions taken for optimal patient care are elicited from content specialists and serve as the basis for the scoring key. This approach was adopted after consideration of and experimentation with other scoring methods, such as analyses of examinee progress at key points in a CBX case or at the end of the case or measuring efficiency in obtaining information.

Expert opinion is obtained for each case prospectively with experts defining criteria for performance before examinees care for the CBX patient. In the ideal situation, perfectly reliable content experts would review each examinee's patient management actions and classify performance as passing or failing. In practice, this would require huge numbers of physicians and would thus be prohibitively expensive and impractical. Great efficiencies are introduced if the computer can perform this review instead of humans. Experts' performance criteria are entered into the computer, compared with examinee performance, and the computer scores candidates on each case accurately, removing one source of rater unreliability.

The goal of CBX scoring is for the computer to rate performance with a result that resembles that produced by expert physician judges, but with reasonable cost and speed in reporting scores. The following section describes the processes by which the computer emulates expert physician scoring.

Input to Scoring

CBX cases provide a rich source of examinee performance information, including sequencing and prioritization of patient care decisions. A record of these decisions is maintained as a *CBX transaction list.* When the case is completed, the CBX transaction list is an accurate, detailed audit trail of the step-by-step decisions made by the examinee managing the CBX patient.

An example of a transaction list is shown in Figure 1. The left column lists the simulated time at which the examinee initiated the action. The far right column lists the simulated time at which a result was seen by the examinee. For example, the CBC with differential was ordered on Day 1 at 10:35 am (beginning of line in figure). The examinee did not see the result until Day 2 at 10:35 am (end of line in figure). The sequence of decisions made by this examinee are revealed by noting actions ordered following results received sequentially over time.

Figure 1. CASE TRANSACTION LIST

Examinee ID: 123-45-6789 Case ID: 77 Date: 11/10/93

Ordered Action Day Hour		Seen Day Hour
1 @ 10:00	History, comprehensive	1 @ 10:20
1 @ 10:20	Physical exam, complete	1 @ 10:35
1 @ 10:35	Cholesterol, serum	1 @ 18:35
1 @ 10:35	Electrocardiography, 12 lead	1 @ 11:05
1 @ 10:35	Chemistry profile 12	1 @ 13:05
1 @ 10:35	CBC with differential	2 @ 10:35
1 @ 10:35	Chemistry profile 6	1 @ 13:05
1 @ 10:35	Skin test, tuberculin	Case ended before result seen
1 @ 10:35	Abstain from alcohol	
1 @ 10:35	No smoking	
1 @ 11:05	Location change to home	
1 @ 11:05	Consult, psychiatry	2 @ 11:05
2 @ 10:35		
2 @ 19:00	History, interval/follow up	2 @ 19:05
2 @ 19:05	Location change to inpatient ward	
2 @ 19:05	Cardiac monitor	2 @ 19:05
2 @ 19:05	Pacemaker, permanent	
2 @ 19:05	History, interval/follow up	2 @ 19:18
2 @ 19:05	Temperature	2 @ 19:18
2 @ 19:05	General appearance	2 @ 19:18
2 @ 19:05	Cardiac examination	2 @ 19:18
2 @ 19:05	Extremities examination	2 @ 19:18
2 @ 19:05	Neurologic/psych examination	2 @ 19:18
2 @ 19:05	Vital signs (MD recorded)	2 @ 19:18
2 @ 19:05	Cardiac monitor	Case ended before result seen
2 @ 21:05	Case end	

Scoring Key

The scoring key contains criteria for performance on a CBX case. It reduces the transaction list to a string of numbers representing the examinee's observed response to the test "questions;" this reduction is the first step in scoring.

A scoring key is produced by a group of expert physicians who manage the CBX case as a group without prior knowledge of the case. They manage the patient as if they were examinees. The content experts represent the broad range of primary care physicians in general medicine. These expert physicians meet in groups of six, and discuss the patient's problem, reviewing alternate approaches to the care of the patient. Once they reach a consensus on appropriate approaches to caring for the CBX patient case, the actions are classified as follows:

Benefit:	Appropriate for patient care distinguishes better examinees from less effective examinees.
Inappropriate:	Not indicated, but not harmful.
Risk:	Poses some probability of harm.
Flag:	Shows the examinee missed the measurement objective of the case or otherwise subjects the patient to unacceptable, and perhaps lethal risk.

Scoring items are defined based on the relative merit, timing, and/or sequence of actions the examinee requested. For example, an examinee might be required simply to order an action (e.g., abdominal ultrasound) and achieve a +1 score for it. Or, the content experts might specify that an abdominal ultrasound (+2) is better than an abdominal x-ray (+1). The examinee ordering the ultrasound would achieve a higher item score than an examinee ordering an x-ray. Action combinations can also be analyzed for scoring. For example, action sequences (if blood cultures ordered **before** antibiotics, score +1; if blood cultures ordered **after** antibiotics, score 0), and timing (if abdominal ultrasound ordered in the first hour, score +2; if ordered after the first hour, score +1) can be defined also. More complex items are possible combining these in any logical way. For an item to be used, there must be consensus by the committee that these definitions comply with their expectations for case performance.

Actions classified in this way represent the "items" on a CBX test. The approach to aggregating these item responses to produce a score that validly represents the examinee's performance has undergone considerable evolution. Early efforts to score CBX demonstrated that a reasonable score could be produced by simply summing the beneficial actions ordered and subtracting from this sum the total number of non-indicated actions. This approach was improved by accounting for the variation in item difficulty by calibrating items using the Rasch (item response theory) model and by allowing for partial credit (based on the timing of the action of other item-related considerations).

Although this score had demonstrated validity, it had the limitation that it disregarded the relative importance of the various item types. The most critical and most trivial actions had the same weight. Subsequently, two approaches to scoring have been developed in an explicit attempt to capture the judgment policy used by experts in rating examinee performance. The first of these utilized a regression-based, policy-capturing procedure.[2] Weights for the various item types were estimated by using expert ratings of transaction lists as the dependent measure and count of items in each category (i.e., inappropriates, risks, benefits, etc.) as the independent measures in a regression equation. The estimated regression weights were then used to weight items to compute scores. The resulting score was shown to be both more highly correlated with the actual ratings than were the previously used scores and to be superior in discriminating between examinees displaying passing and failing performance based on independent judgment of the performance.[2]

This line of research demonstrated that a more valid score could be produced by weighting items based on the relative importance of the actions. The limitation of this approach was that it failed to account fully for the possible interaction of actions in the process of managing a case. For example, two diagnostic procedures may provide important but redundant information and using a statistical actuarial approach to scoring may result in some examinees receiving inflated scores. To address this limitation, more recent research has focused on attempting to relate scores directly to patterns of behavior. Again, the approach involves capturing the policy decisions used by experts in judging (rating) transaction lists. This approach avoids the need to base scores on a sum of items, weighted or otherwise, and avoids the possibility of rewarding redundancy. Rewarding thoroughness over efficiency has been a long-standing problem in scoring clinical simulations.

This most recent approach to scoring also has other important advantages. The approach is substantive (i.e., based on the structure of the case) rather than actuarial (i.e., based on estimates of characteristics of a population) and is largely independent of the sample of examinees who completed the test. As a result, the scoring system should be invariant across potential populations of examinees. Also, the scoring algorithm can be developed prior to test administration, a substantial advantage for nearly immediate reporting of scores.

Research on the performance of this "substantive" approach to scoring shows that, similar to the regression-based procedure, it produces a result that is more highly correlated to the actual ratings compared to earlier scoring methods; and it is substantially more useful than the earlier scores in discriminating between examinees' performances that are judged passing or failing as defined independently by experts.

Standard Setting

In standard setting, physician content experts decide how to separate passing from failing performance. Different methods have been reviewed and tested with committees to demonstrate that a workable and effective technique is available. For example, in one exercise physician experts reviewed transaction lists, independently judging each performance as passing or failing. Discrepancies were then discussed by the group individually and judges were given an opportunity to change their decisions. The results showed that distributions of performances judged as passing and those judged as failing were largely non-overlapping across the scale produced by the weighted scores. This type of contrasting group data provides an appropriate basis for identifying a cut score.[3] In addition to group decisions showing clear separation of passing and failing performances across the score scale, the high level of reported inter-judge agreement argues for the procedure's replicability.[3]

On examination-level standard setting, preliminary work suggests that expert physicians use a less than fully "compensatory" approach. The physicians tend not to allow acceptable performance on one case to offset unacceptable performance on another. The physicians tend to say, "If you killed three patients out of eight, it doesn't matter how you managed the other five." Research is continuing to find effective ways to implement this judgment strategy in making examination level pass/fail decisions.

Is CBX Valid?

CBX is intended for licensure decisions of future physicians. The validity of CBX cases can be evaluated by examining test content, score characteristics, and construct-related evidence.

Content Expertise

One part of the foundation for claims about the validity for CBX cases is the expertise of case, scoring key, and standard-setting committee members. Content experts refine the features of individual case simulations; they specify the competencies, problems, and diagnoses to be tested; they select sets of patient problems that best meet defined test objectives; they define how patient problems will unfold based on examinee intervention; their collective judgment on patient management strategies is used to build scoring criteria; they interpret examinee performance as part of key validation; their judgment policies are used to determine item weighting and ultimately the rank ordering of examinees; and their judgment is emulated in setting pass/fail standards at both case and examination levels.

Training Level Performance Cmparisons

Comparisons of performance at different levels of training have shown that physicians more advanced in training achieve higher scores than physicians not as advanced in training. In a study conducted in 1987, the performance of 73 third-year medical students and 202 first-year residents was significantly different after adjusting for covariates (the resident group was generally more able than the student group after adjusting for differences in MCAT and NBME Part I scores).[4]

Comparison With Other Measures of Knowledge and Performance

Comparisons with MCQs show correlations between .35 and .55 (corrected for unreliability of both exam formats). This could be interpreted in many ways. It suggests that CBX and MCQ examinations measure related constructs; however, different examinees are identified for failure by the two formats. Comparisons have not yet been made to characterize examinees who fail one format and pass the other.

By far the strongest argument in support of the validity of CBX measures is the fact that CBX scoring emulates physician judgment of examinee performance. The foundation underlying this assertion is that the simulation is a good depiction of features central to physicians' professional tasks, and that it elicits and records behaviors like those physicians manifest in real life. That performance is scored by a proxy for expert judges. Expert judges are deemed to be the best "gold standard" available for comparison. That CBX scores are modeled after, and closely emulate expert judgment of CBX performance, means that CBX will score automatically examinees with a result similar to that produced by expert judges.

Other Factors

Studies to date have shown that computer experience, computer anxiety, and gender do not show a systematic influence on performance measures obtained using CBX cases. There is, however, a need for examinees to practice with CBX cases before being tested. This effect may require practice on three to four CBX cases to ensure sufficient familiarity with the software.[4,5]

Is CBX Reliable?

Examination results should be reproducible so that the measures are a stable estimate of a person's ability. More importantly, it is vital that the margin of error in the score is as small as possible at the point from which a decision must be made about examinee performance (i.e., pass/fail etc.). Performance assessments, like CBX, require more examinee time than traditional written tests using MCQs, for example. The measure of reliability or accuracy at the pass-fail point for any test is dependent in large part on the number of items (or cases for CBX) encountered by the examinee. Because each CBX case is complex (compared with an MCQ), it requires more time on an item by item basis. To approach the accuracy of MCQ tests, CBX requires more time. To achieve acceptable accuracy, a CBX examination may require from eight to 16 simulations depending on the content area assessed and the intended use of the measures. This represents from 4-8 hours of testing time.

Is Nationwide Administration Feasible?

The National Board of Medical Examiners has five years' experience with use of CBX in medical schools in the United States and Canada. About half the schools have used sets of cases in a non-testing setting. A subset of those schools has used CBX to assess students in clinical clerkships. Some schools have the available resources to administer CBX; others do not. While facilities within schools are commonly adequate for testing, the lack of standardization of facilities across schools raises questions of comparability of test environments and security of test materials. Greater standardization of facilities will likely be required for CBX use in licensure assessment. Standardized facilities have been developed by commercial vendors and are already being used nationally to administer licensure and aptitude examinations. In these facilities, careful attention has been paid to security of the testing system.

What is the Plan for Use of CBX?

Prototype examinations are being developed for use in intramural assessment. One examination is comprehensive and interdisciplinary intended for assessment of medical students at the conclusion of medical school (after core clinical rotations are completed). Another is an internal medicine subject examination intended for end of clerkship evaluation. The subject examination will serve as a prototype for other discipline-based subject examinations. Market surveys have been conducted to assess medical schools' readiness for use of CBX for medical student intramural assessment and demonstrate a perceived need for and interest in additional assessment services.

The NBME and the Federation of State Medical Boards, as parents of the United States Medical Licensure Examination (USMLE) program, have recently endorsed a plan for implementing CBX in USMLE Step 3. Implementation planning is now underway, with specific timing of the implementation not yet determined.

References

1. Consensus Statement of the Researchers in Clinical Skills Assessment (RSCA) on the Use of Standardized Patients to Evaluate Clinical Skills. *Acad Med* 1993; 68:475.

2. Clauser BE, Subhiyah R, Nungester RJ, Ripkey DR, Clyman SG, McKinley D. Scoring a performance-based assessment by modeling the judgments of experts. *J Educ Meas* (In press).

3. Clauser BE, Clyman SG. A contrasting group's approach to standard setting for performance assessments of clinical skills. *Proceedings Acad Med* 1994; 69:S42-S44.

4. *Proceedings* Conference on Computer-Based Testing in Medical Education and Evaluation - *March 24, 1988*. National Board of Medical Examiners, Philadelphia.

5. *Interim Report* CBT Phase II. National Board of Medical Examiners, Philadelphia. October 1990.

Recommended Reading

Clauser BE, Ross PL, et al. Development of a scoring algorithm to replace expert rating for scoring a complex performance-based assessment. Paper presented at the Ann Meet Nat Council Measurement Educ, San Francisco, CA April 18-22, 1995. (Unpublished manuscript).

Messick S. The Interplay of Evidence and Consequences in the Validation of Performance Assessment. *Research Report RR-92-39* Princeton, NJ: Educational Testing Service, 1992.

Moss PA. Shifting Conceptions of Validity in Educational Measurement. *Rev Educ Res* 1992; 62:229-258.

National Board of Medical Examiners' Computer-Based Examination Clinical Simulation (CBX). National Board of Medical Examiners, Philadelphia, PA. Spring 1991.

Swanson DB, Norcini JJ, Gross J. Assessment of clinical competence: written and computer-based simulations. *Assess Eval Higher Educ* 1987; 12:220-246.

Inter-Station Progress Notes

Paula L. Stillman, M.D.
Medical College of Pennsylvania

Youde Wang, Ph.D.
Eastern Virginia Medical School

Alfred E. Stillman, M.D.
Crozer Chester Hospital, Upland, PA

Although there is a wealth of literature on teaching and assessment of clinical problem solving, there does not seem to be agreement on a single method that has proven both reliable and valid. The use of standardized patients (SPs) to assess clinical skills of medical students has been adopted in many medical schools. Content checklists filled out by SPs or observers after each encounter provide a wealth of information about an examinee's skills in obtaining the medical history, performing the physical examination, communicating with patients, and possibly, generating some initial diagnosis and treatment plans. Close examination of this methodology, however, reveals that certain critical pieces of information, such as clinical reasoning or interpretation of information and decision making, are not readily assessed. For example, the SP or observer can tell if an examinee listened to the heart in the correct locations, if both the bell and diaphragm of the stethoscope were used, and if appropriate pressure was applied. The SP or observer cannot determine, however, what the examinee heard, if normal was distinguished from abnormal, if the findings were interpreted correctly, and if an appropriate diagnosis was generated. In other words, clinical reasoning or problem solving is different from performing a series of actions, such as obtaining a chief complaint or measuring blood pressure, which can be recorded by a checklist. Clinical reasoning should be evaluated in a way, we believe, that documents the logical reasoning of an examinee. This type of information combined with the information obtained from checklists may provide us with a more complete picture of an examinee's clinical skills.

Over the past twenty-five years we have used various formats of post-encounter paperwork following SP encounters to assess clinical reasoning. We believe that clinical reasoning is difficult to define clearly but at a minimum involves:

Collection of appropriate and relevant information.
Interpretation of information.
Synthesis of information into an initial differential diagnosis and
Collection of additional information from the results of diagnostic studies to confirm or refute the differential diagnosis.

The above steps may need to be repeated several times.

One of the methods we have used to assess clinical reasoning following SP encounters is multiple choice questions (MCQs). Queries about medical history, physical examination, diagnosis and management plans were developed using an MCQ format. While MCQs are easy to score, they provide a significant degree of cuing and seem to favor those examinees with better test-taking skills. Another format we used consisted of presentation of a series of possible diagnoses, asking the examinee to indicate if each was most likely, possible, or unlikely. We have used a similar format for prioritizing initial plans. In both instances, however, it was difficult to get a group of experts to agree on the answer keys.

More recently, we have developed a format that has minimal cuing and approximates the real-life task a physician performs in his or her office. We call this strategy "patient notes." Immediately following the encounter, each examinee is given seven minutes to construct a patient note. The note is almost uncued, we ask the examinee to (1) document the subjective findings (include chief complaint, and significant positives and negatives from history of present illness, past medical history, review of systems, social history and family history); (2) record the objective findings (include only pertinent positive and negative findings related to patient's chief complaint); (3) list possible initial differential diagnoses (prioritize and include no more than three diagnostic hypotheses); and (4) formulate management plans (immediate plan for further diagnostic workup and possible treatment; i.e., only include plans to be initiated today). This approach was first used in 1989 for fourth-year medical students from several schools in New England participating in a graduation clinical skills examination. The authors of each case developed a list of key words or phrases that should be included in each of the sections. These were listed in a checklist format on a scannable form. On average, each case contained about 25 items.

Record-room clerks were recruited and trained for about 45 minutes by a physician to review the handwritten patient notes and document the presence of the key words and phrases. Eight clerks were recruited; each was assigned one case. On average, 20 notes could be scored each hour. To check the scorers' accuracy, a subset of notes was also scored by a physician (PLS). The correlations between physicians and non-physicians ranged from 0.81 to 0.98 for the eight cases, with an overall correlation of 0.90.

These same SP cases and key words and phrases for patient notes were later used as part of the clinical skills project of the Educational Commission for Foreign Medical Graduates (ECFMG). We wanted to explore the relationship between data obtained from patient notes as compared to MCQs. Two hundred sixty-five examinees completed the patient notes following each of eight SP encounters and immediately thereafter were asked to respond to several MCQs about the patient's diagnosis. On average, fifty-eight percent of examinees (range from 38 to 91) reported correct diagnosis on the uncued patient notes and seventy-seven percent of examinees (range from 61 to 94) chose the correct diagnosis on the cued MCQ format ($p<.05$). It was not uncommon for an examinee to fail to list the correct diagnosis on the patient note but then chose it when it was presented on the cued MCQ format. The discrepancy between patient notes and MCQs in obtaining a correct diagnosis suggests that a cued format tends to overestimate a significant number of examinees' diagnostic skills. The free-response format may yield a more accurate measure of examinees' clinical skills and have high fidelity to the real-life tasks performed by a physician.[1]

Although it seemed feasible to use non-physicians to document examinees' clinical skills using the key words or phrases as noted above, it soon became clear to the physician reading the same notes that the record clerks were not able to detect false positive or false negative findings. Further, non-physicians could not judge the relevance of the differential diagnosis or estimate how closely it reflected the recorded information, or assess the appropriateness of the initial diagnostic and management plans. The clerks could tell if specific key words and phrases were listed but had no way to detect items that were inappropriate, overly expensive, or dangerous. This level of differentiation requires the clinical skills of a physician.

In light of these issues, we decided to assess in another investigation how closely a physician's rating of the patient notes using criteria employed in actual clinical settings would correlate with the scoring of a non-physician. If the correlations were high, we could be more secure in allowing the scoring to be done by non-physicians and would feel satisfied that the data captured by searching for key words and phrases were sufficient to present a true appraisal of the examinee's skills. If the correlations were low, we would have to conclude that despite the time and cost involved, only physicians could score the handwritten patient notes.

Rather than using key words and phrases, we developed a more global rating scale for the physicians to use. It included the following categories:

Clarity (readability, precision of language, neatness).

Organization (logical, focused, internally consistent).

Accuracy (complete, concise, relevant, no errors of omission or commission).

Analysis (synthesis, differential diagnosis appropriate for data collected).

Management (appropriate for current resolution of the problem).

Each item was rated on a five point scale, with five representing excellent, three representing competent and one representing poor. A representative sample of 10 cases and 204 patient notes scored by both physicians and non-physicians was used for analysis. The physicians read a summary of each SP case, and on average could score 20 notes within one hour.

Correlations between patient notes scores generated by physicians and non-physicians are displayed in Table 1. They range from 0.21 to 0.64, indicating a moderate correlation. Reliability coefficients for physicians and non-physicians are almost identical.

Table 1. Correlations Between Patient Notes Scored by Physicians and Record Room Clerks

SP-Case	R-Values	P-Values
Headaches	0.21	0.37
RUQ Pain	0.46	0.04
Confusion	0.64	0.002
Female Chest Pain	0.53	0.01
Male Chest Pain	0.44	0.06
Weight Loss, Polyuria	0.51	0.02
Low Back Pain	0.24	0.31
Panic Attack	0.32	0.16
Fatigue (Alcohol)	0.39	0.09
RLQ Pain	0.51	0.02

Cronbach Coefficient Alpha	
Physician	.62
Non-Physician	.61

Although there is a reasonable correlation between a non-physician's rating of key words and phrases and a physician's more global rating, there is added value when the physician reads the patient notes. A physician is able to detect inconsistencies, false/positive findings, and errors of omission and commission of the differential diagnosis and initial plan. He or she is also able to evaluate sloppy and imprecise recording practices. A non-physician may assign a zero score to an examinee if his/her diagnosis does not match the key words or phrases, without knowing or understanding the cause of difficulty. A physician might identify the reasons why examinees missed the diagnosis. For example, examinees often had difficulties in cases involving substance abuse and psychological problems. For those two cases, the patient's problems were often diagnosed as occult malignancies or "anemia." This was obvious to the physician rater who noted that important information from the patient's history was not obtained, or was ignored or misinterpreted. Another example, several examinees recorded that there was no past history of surgery on a patient who had a clearly visible scar from a cholecystectomy. In addition, a physician was able to detect large inconsistencies in patient notes when several examinees created a written record on the same SP. It is possible that the SP provided a different story to each examinee, but this is unlikely because all the SPs involved in this project were well-trained and experienced subjects.

Because the SP station is usually fixed in time, however, it is difficult to use the results of follow-up information to modify the initial diagnosis and plan. This can be artificially accomplished with a sequential type of simulation where the "clock advances" and the examinee is allowed to act at a "later time period."

In conclusion, it is possible to evaluate clinical reasoning or problem-solving using post-encounter patient notes in a free response format. Since patient notes provide essentially no cuing and represent the real-life tasks performed by a physician, patient notes can serve as a realistic assessment of the examinees' clinical reasoning.

We believe that the patient notes are a promising technique for evaluating clinical reasoning and problem-solving skills. Additional research is required to establish more structured scoring criteria. Inter-rater and intra-rater reliabilities of physician scoring also need to be examined.

References

1. Stillman PL, Reagan MB, Haley HA, Norcini JJ, Friedman M, Sutnick AI. The use of a patient note to evaluate clinical skills of first-year residents who are graduates of foreign medical schools. *Acad Med* 1992; 67:S57-S59.

The Canadian Oral Examination

Jacques E. Des Marchais, M.D.
Université de Sherbrooke

The Royal College of Physicians and Surgeons of Canada (The Royal College) recently reviewed its evaluation system for specialist certification. Assessing clinical reasoning remains a necessary component of the certification examination for specialists in Canada. Examiners continue to prefer the traditional oral examination.[1,2]

Why do clinicians insist so much on retaining this evaluation format? Is it only to control those who would join a private club of specialists? Many argue that it is essential to measure clinical reasoning through modalities closer to "real world" situations. The process of "thinking aloud" inherent in the orals and so useful to cognitive psychologists provides considerable although only face validity. While we do not boast that Canadians have a perfect oral examination, this paper is intended to demonstrate how the Royal College uses oral examinations, and to describe the questioning patterns of oral examiners as analyzed in a research project carried out a few years ago.

Royal College Oral Examinations Leading to Certification

The Royal College is responsible for certifying the competence of physicians prior to being recognized as specialists in Canada. Since 1969, the Royal College evaluation system has benefited from the educational resources of the R.S. McLaughlin Research and Examination Center that became later the McLaughlin Center for Evaluation.

In 1972, the in-training evaluation system was introduced as a progressive in-service type of resident assessment. In the last decade, the evaluation process has been improved by the application of model answers and marking schemes to written and oral examinations, in order to promote fairness and objectivity. In 1990, the comprehensive objective examination based on a clear definition of the daily tasks of a specialist, was introduced in a few specialties, some using the OSCE format (Objective Structured Clinical Encounter, a multi-station practical examination) format along with other assessment formats.

While these developments were taking place, great variability among specialties, escalating costs, and extensive costly evaluation procedures for some subspecialties have led the Evaluation Committee to reexamine its operation. In 1992/1993 a special task force was established to study the College's evaluation system. Although many of its recommendations remain to be implemented by examination boards and specialty committees, the traditional examination is undergoing rapid evolution.

As of 1994, thirty-nine of the forty-three specialties recognized by the Royal College have continued to use an oral examination for the certification process. The oral examination sessions last from one to three hours. Each year approximately 1200 candidates are assessed by about 800 clinical examiners.

Oral examinations may take various shapes according to the specialty. For instance, in internal medicine the examination is "designed to measure the clinical competence of the candidate to function in a consultant role." Assessed are the mastery of such skills as history taking, physical examination, interpretation of laboratory tests data, the ability to process information rapidly and coherently, and to formulate a sensible course of investigation and treatment. The examination consists of a long and a short clinical case, each involving two different examiners and including physical examination questions and clinical problem-solving exercises, all of which are standardized. In orthopaedic surgery, by comparison, candidates are assessed by two different teams of three examiners, one team dealing with pediatrics and the relevant basic sciences, the other with reconstructive surgery, trauma, and surgical sciences. The examination is patient-oriented and problem-based.

Even though the assessment models seem to be quite traditional, a few specialties began developing the Comprehensive Objective Examination (COE) in 1990. The COE is a "summative examination based on learning objectives, utilizing various appropriate assessment instruments, and intended to certify the competence of residents upon entering a professional career in a medical, a surgical, or a non-clinical specialty." It is intended to maximize relevance and minimize obvious bias. It too varies from specialty to specialty, not only in content, but also in process and in method as dictated by the objectives to be measured. By and large, as already pointed out, the COE uses the OSCE format with standardized patients and standardized orals. Proponents of the COE argue that it has the following advantages:

1. Fits the examination methods to the objective. However, the multi-station examinations are excellent but not necessarily the best instrument for all the objectives; traditional examinations have their own rationale and have been retained for many sets of objectives.
2. Measures previously untested objectives, for instance, communications skills.
3. Achieves content validity with the appearance of realism, as well as predicting more accurately future performance.
4. Uses simple situations and problems to obtain an examination of good quality by avoiding excessively complex measurement items, such as long, exhaustive check lists. It is most important to have clear objectives, to measure them well, and to set reasonable criteria for performance.
5. Moves the examination process toward criterion-referenced standard setting, mainly reached by consensus for a predetermined level of performance.
6. Increases the expertise for the Royal College examiners. The development and introduction of COE has exerted a powerful "Hawthorne effect" on examiners, causing them to acquire further educational skills and to reconsider traditional examination methods.

Thus, the Royal College examinations are becoming more specialty-specific, more objective, more comprehensive, and we hope, more valid.

So far, six specialties (diagnostic radiology, medical genetics, obstetrics and gynecology, physical medicine and rehabilitation, urology, and general and anatomical pathology) have developed their comprehensive objective examination in the new format, including an oral examination component. A moratorium on further extension of the method is presently in effect because of cost constraints.

In developing a COE, a specialty board must carry out the following tasks in order to ensure content validity: 1) define the professional tasks of the practicing specialist, 2) define the educational domain corresponding to those tasks, and 3) define the objectives to be evaluated. OSCE stations may be developed to measure clinically relevant content with acceptable standards of performance established a priori. In this manner, several components of clinical competence can be assessed through a variety of examination formats, including standardized patients and structured orals.

Four out of the six specialties have integrated standardized patient encounters, typically associated with OSCE stations. All six have a structured oral examination and assess closely related professional tasks using simulated cases with assessment of visual recognition and/or consultation. Table 1 describes the variety of OSCE station formats used by the six specialties.

Table 1. Types of OSCE* Stations by Specialty

Type of Station / Specialty	Standardized Patient Encounter	Structured Oral	Visual Recognition	Consultation
Diagnostic Radiology		x	x	x
Medical Genetics	x	x	x	x
Obstetrics & Gynecology	x	x	x	x
Physical Medicine & Rehabilitation	x	x	x	x
Urology	x	x	x	x
Anatomical Pathology & General Pathology		x	x	

*Objective Structured Clinical Encounter

The development and implementation of COEs is seen by many as a major advance in the assessment of clinical competence. This model is to be extended to other specialties after the completion and evaluation of the present pilot project, including psychometric analyses and cost-benefit assessments.

In the OSCE-type format, errors of measurement can stem from many sources because of the many types of measurement involved, the limited number of raters and stations. To assess reliability of these multi-method, multi-situation examination formats a generalizability theory is being used to identify which statistically potential sources of variability account for measurement error. This analysis should help to identify and determine what is needed to attain an acceptable degree of exam reliability and measurement.

The Royal College evaluation system for specialist certification relies upon examination boards in each of forty-three specialties. The examination boards are accountable to the evaluation committee, and with their specialty committees who oversee the testing activities, are directly in touch with the Board of Directors of the Royal College (see Figure 1). Each examination board is responsible for all examinations leading to certification in the specialty, with assistance from the McLaughlin Centre for Evaluation. The system can be compared to a fleet of many ships, each having its own crew and course with the captain and the sailors generally confident that they know what is good or bad for them.

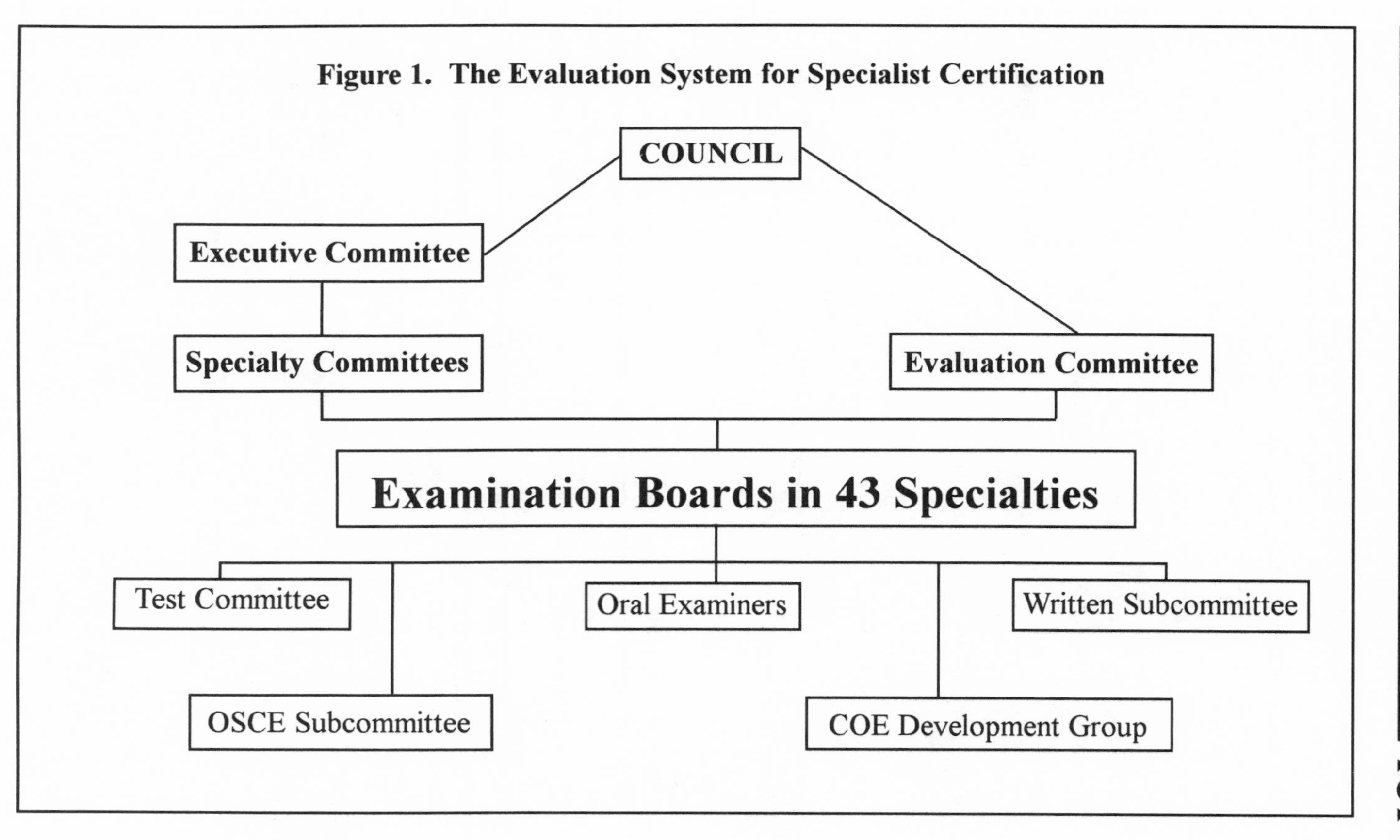

Figure 1. The Evaluation System for Specialist Certification

In 1992, a special task force was given the mandate to study the examination system of the Royal College. It made recommendations to the evaluation committee and were subsequently accepted by the Council in September 1993.[3] All 25 recommendations were to be implemented through the regular procedures of the evaluation committee and the McLaughlin Centre for Evaluation.

Regarding the oral examinations, the task force recommended that:

1) All examination boards justify their need to retain or introduce the oral format in relation to specific measurement objectives.
2) Several clinical scenarios be used instead of one or two long cases.
3) Examinations become more objective and standardized in a given specialty, so that content and process are predetermined and relevant to the learning objectives.
4) Examiners work independently, allowing a large number of scenarios to be tested.

With respect to examiners, the task force recommended the examiners be offered opportunities to become proficient in evaluation techniques, particularly in the art of questioning, and that examiner performance should be monitored periodically. Those recommendations are relevant to the reality of many oral examinations because they retain for the time being a very traditional profile.

Questioning Patterns of Oral Examiners

The effect of training on the questioning patterns of oral examiners, specifically their ability to raise open-ended and high-taxonomic level questions (lowest is single recall, next data interpretation, and highest problem-solving), were studied for the Royal College's oral examinations in orthopaedics.[4]

The study proceeded in four phases over a period of five years.

Table 2. Oral Certification Examinations*

	Examiners				
Phase	Untrained	Trained	Candidates	Problems	Questions
I	5	–	2	25	334
II	–	7	12	101	1,349
III	5	8	18	150	2,334
IV	10	7	15	105	1,773
Total	20	22	47	381	5,790

*From Des Marchais JE, Jean P. - Teach & Learn Med 1993; 5:24-28

In Phase I, an observational study recorded the number of open-ended and closed-ended questions asked by a group of 5 French-speaking examiners. The following year in Phase II, 7 French-speaking examiners were observed after being taught how to ask open-ended questions at higher taxonomic levels. In Phase III, the experiment was extended to train half of the English-speaking examiners during a three-hour training session before the examination. Two years later, in Phase IV, both groups of English and French examiners, some previously trained and others untrained, were observed again.

Thus, the performance of 20 untrained examiners was compared to that of 22 trained examiners, during examinations in which 47 candidates were assessed over 381 problems. Each of the 5790 questions asked at these orals was scored as to whether it was closed or open-ended, and whether the question was at one of three taxonomic levels; simple recall, interpretation of data, or problem-solving.[5]

The training period was somewhat uncomplicated. The day before the examination, examiners were trained by three medical educators in the art of asking open-ended questions of high taxonomic levels. The objective was clearly to change the questioning behavior of examiners from the close-ended and recall pattern demonstrated in the pilot phase. The three-hour training workshop involved participants in scoring and classifying 10 questions by taxonomic level. In the second exercise, examinees were asked to distinguish closed- from open-ended questions. They were later asked to consider correct practical answers for questions which were problem-solving, evaluation, or judgment. The consensus method of group decision making by groups of three was used with the examination cases, each participant had the opportunity to generate questions, to receive feedback from peer examiners, and to correct errors.

An important difference between trained and untrained examiners was apparent in the percentage of open-ended questions and those involving the problem-solving level of questioning. (See Figure 2.)

Combining the four studies together, it was found that trained examiners asked 60% open-ended questions in comparison to 45% for untrained examiners, and 49% questions at the problem-solving taxonomic level in comparison to 34% without training. These results support the original hypothesis that without adequate training, examiners are ill-prepared and unable to generate adequate open-ended questions at the problem-solving taxonomic level. Many have had the same experience in oral examinations. Without training, the clinician tends to reproduce the familiar pattern of an MCQ-type examination, as documented long ago in the literature,[6] and still apparent in today's examination systems. Training helps examiners to ask more open-ended questions and raise their taxonomic level, as shown in this study.

Another finding from the study was that the percentage of problem-solving questions remained nearly constant on average throughout the four half-days of the oral examination session. (See Table 3).

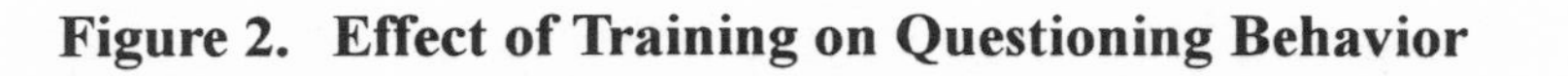

Figure 2. Effect of Training on Questioning Behavior

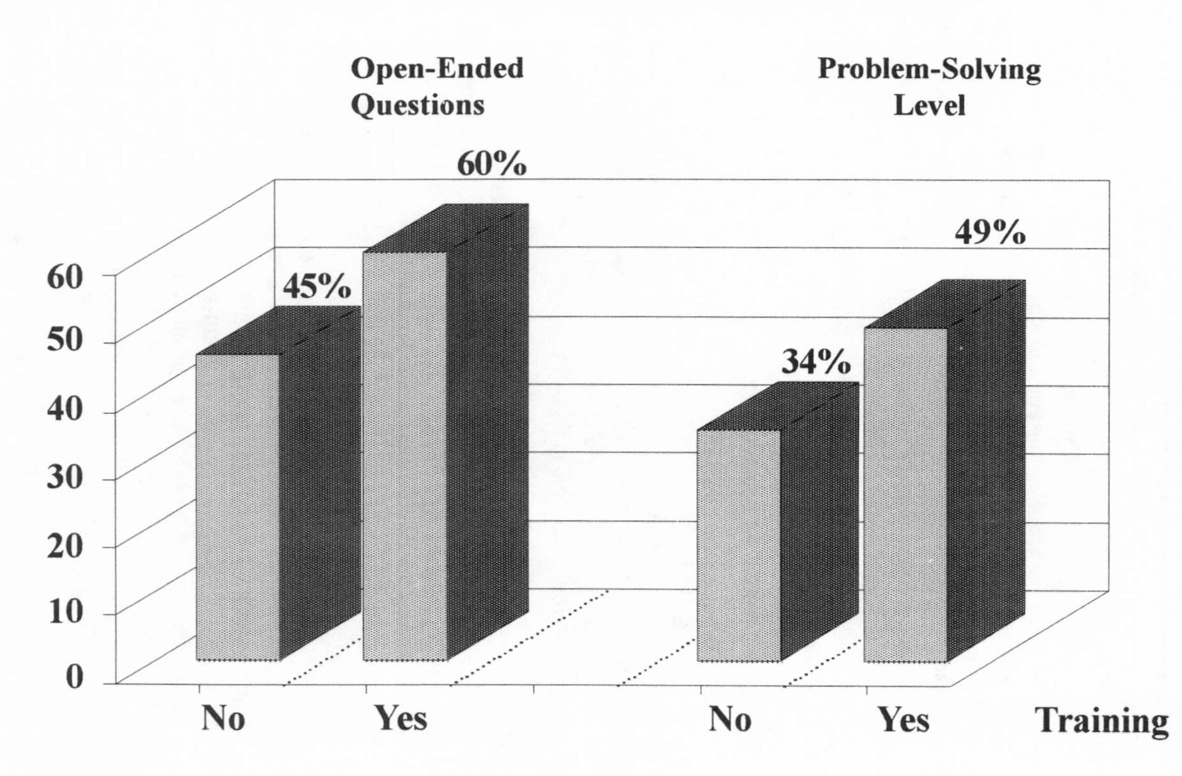

Table 3.

PERCENTAGE OF PROBLEM-SOLVING QUESTIONS OVER FOUR HALF-DAY EXAMINATION SESSIONS (2 DAYS)

	EXAMINATION SESSIONS			
Phases	**First**	**Second**	**Third**	**Fourth**
I	21	21	--	--
II	35	47	41	--
III	42	55	55	55
IV	46	44	52	47

This suggests that examiners learn and change their behavior in the first session, and maintain the change over subsequent examination. Thus, there was a sustained learning effect throughout subsequent examinations in the experiment. From these studies, we may draw the following conclusions:

- A three-hour training workshop for examiners can increase the percentage of problem-solving questions used by examination from 20% initially to nearly 50%.
- A three-hour training session can have a lasting effect on the questioning behavior of examiners for the orthopaedic surgery examination board.
- The change in questioning behavior is maintained throughout the examination session over a 2-day period. Even without reinforcement through further training, the questioning behavior is still present two years later. There was also an impact on the untrained examiners, a nice illustration of the "contaminating" effect of an experiment.
- The use of open-ended questions at the problem-solving level improves the content validity of oral examination, at least from a qualitative aspect. This type of questioning better assesses what the oral examination is intended to assess in the first place—a candidate's problem-solving ability and sound clinical reasoning.

Conclusion

In conclusion, anyone with experience as an oral examiner and as an instructor of examiners, and aware of the recommendations on the evaluation system for specialist certification, must return to the basics of any educational program. As with other programs, a residency program must contain three major components. **Identified learning** needs and **learning objectives** must be formulated and correlated with specific clinical rotations, which become the preferred instructional method for learning clinical reasoning. The third component is the **evaluation of the competencies** acquired and of the specialty skills and abilities mastered. The conclusion is very simple. The evaluation system must be guided by sound educational and psychometric principles, which leads us in turn to the conclusion of the task force report on the evaluation system: "Now, the challenge lies not in deciding what we must do, but in convincing all of us that we **can** do what **must** be done."[3]

The Royal College Task Force deliberations and the preparation of the report on the evaluation system for specialists certification took place in a climate of exceptional thoroughness and broadmindedness, in spite of the multitude of concerns identified by the stakeholders of the evaluation system. A consensus had developed on the necessary improvements that will be valid, reliable, economically feasible, and acceptable to the 43 specialties and subspecialties for which certificates are granted, their subcommittees and the many hundreds of Fellows who are responsible for the examinations. Although all specialties and subspecialties are rightfully jealous of their individuality, many commonalities were evident with respect to the assessment of clinical competence. The recommendations were seen as congruent with current advances in educational evaluation and measurement, and with the degree of cost-effectiveness and financial responsibility expected by the residents and by Council.

The author is indebted to Dr. Bernard-M. Lefebvre, Director of the McLaughin Center for Evaluation for his advice and editorial assistance.

References

1. Foster JT, Abrahamson S, Lass S, Girard R, Garris R. Analysis of an oral examination used in specialty board certification. *J Med Educ* 1969; 44:951-954.

2. Pokorny AD, Frazier SH. An evaluation of oral examinations. *J Med Educ* 1966; 41:28-40.

3. Des Marchais JE and Task Force Members. *Report on the Evaluation System for Specialist Certification. Evaluation Committee.* The Royal College of Physicians and Surgeons of Canada, Ottawa, July 1993.

4. Des Marchais JE, Jean P. Effects of examiner training on open-ended, high taxonomic level questioning in oral certification examinations. *Teach & Learn Med* 1993; 5(1):24-28.

5. McGuire CH. In JJ Guilbert (Ed.) *Educational Handbook for Health Personnel* (WHO publication No. 35). Geneva: World Health Organization 1981.

6. McGuire CH. The oral examination as a measure of professional competence. *J Med Educ* 1966; 41:267-274.

Discussion

Dr. John F.W. Kelly (American Board of Oral & Maxillofacial Surgery): I have two questions, one for Dr. Dauphinee and one for Dr. Clyman. I would like to come away from this conference knowing how to improve the process of our examination and I am very attracted to the notion of the short answer. I'm curious as to how one gets around the issue of penmanship. Is it really true that the Canadian school system produces better penmanship and makes the scoring possible? Second, for Dr. Clyman, I know that several years ago when I had the pleasure of designing a computer-based (CBX) case it was thought that the methodology was not acceptable for life and death situations, i.e., licensure, but was good for clinical clerkships and nonfatal situations. What has changed in CBX methodology and makes it acceptable now for the life and death situation?

Dr. Stephen G. Clyman (National Board of Medical Examiners): I think the big advance in the last couple of years pertains to scoring simulations. In the past we were not concerned about which action somebody actually undertook. For instance, if the candidate was required to take ten actions appropriately in the simulation, if they did one thing wrong, the scoring systems would then indicate that the performance was good, i.e., nine out of ten, clearly a simplification. It really depends on the identity of the one item wrong out of the ten actions. Previous scoring schema would score both the trivial error and the important mistake as nine out of ten correct. Under the current scoring system,however, physicians score what actions are important actions and actions which must be done, and what actions are less important. It is no longer a simple count of correct actions minus incorrect actions. Rather, the specific actions performed are judged. A major error which could kill the patient would result in failing the candidate, while someone who forgot an unimportant item might still earn a high score. There has thus been a major conceptual change in scoring. We consider it an important advance.

Dr. Mancall: Dr. Dauphinee, did you want to comment on the Canadian experience?

Dr. W. Dale Dauphinee (Medical Council of Canada): With respect to penmanship, scoring is done by young physicians with fine eyesight! Scoring is handled quite well. In the last examination with about 2,200 candidates I would estimate that the Medical Council encountered only a half-a-dozen exams in which it was hard to read the writing; most of those we were able to resolve. Obviously, like everybody else, we are looking forward to using computers in the near future so as to avoid the penmanship problem. Your point is well taken, but it has not turned out to be a big problem, I suspect, because the candidates know it matters and are extra careful.

Professor Christine McGuire (University of Illinois): I am Christine McGuire of the University of Illinois, alleged mentor of Dr. Page, for whom I refuse to accept full credit. I wish to make an observation, ask a question, and enter a plea.

The observation: Dr. Des Marchais has called our attention to the existence of differences in the subcultures of various specialties; I would like to call your attention to important differences in the general culture of medicine over time. As but one example, the views of several of today's speakers make clear that the value attached to "comprehensive" data collection has come full circle in the last 30 years. In the decade before I entered the field some 35 years ago, the Rimoldi Test, though impractical to administer to large numbers of candidates, was greatly admired as a test of clinical judgment. It was analogous to a game of 20 Questions in which the object was to reach the diagnosis as quickly and efficiently as possible. Extensive data gathering was punished. By the time I came along and began to work with the PMP (a form of written simulation of medical decision making) the medical culture (at least in academia) had shifted 180 degrees; the premium was on "comprehensive" data gathering to assure that nothing was being missed as a result of premature closure, and the PMP was deliberately designed and scored to reward compulsive histories and physical examinations—the very characteristics for which it is now being rejected. The techniques described today—key features, CBX, etc.—seem once again to be focused on getting the right diagnosis and making the appropriate interventions—certainly, skills of critical importance in the delivery of patient care. But is that all there is to it?

The question: Should we be concerned that, with their emphasis on "getting the right answer," these newer techniques risk undervaluing the equally important *prerequisite* skills of knowing what data to collect and how to separate important information from noise? Is there a more appropriate middle ground?

The plea: I believe we need once again to examine the demands of real life, identify the essential components of competence, and design our test exercises and scoring systems so as to reward the requisite skills accordingly.

Dr. Jacques E. Des Marchais (Université de Sherbrooke, Quebec): I would be very interested to know the evaluation of the thinking process of physicians because that knowledge would be helpful to improve teaching and learning in medical school. In the last 20 years I have seen a shift toward the institution taking responsibility to develop an internal process of evaluation for medical students as distinguished from the external evaluation by the boards, the Medical Council of Canada, or the Royal College. From the boards' point of view the interest is in the outcome measure, the product of someone's thinking, the professional task or the performance, but the medical school must focus upon learning to think as a physician.

Dr. Dauphinee: Out of our experiences, scoring should be case-centered and not simply concerned with just how much knowledge is possessed. Even with the key features cases we do not punish people for acquiring other important and contributory data. It is possible to resolve the problem of a patient presenting with a headache vis-a-vis a migraine or not, by gathering several different forms of data. The candidate might not even ask the same questions, but come to the correct conclusion and, presumably, then initiate the correct action. So I do not see the two scoring methods as being mutually exclusive.

CERTIFYING PILOTS: IMPLICATIONS FOR MEDICINE AND FOR THE FUTURE

PART 7

Certifying Pilots: Implications for Medicine and for the Future

William R. Taggart
University of Texas at Austin
NASA/UT/FAA Aerospace Crew Research Project

Approximately seventy percent of aviation accidents have "human factors" as one of the contributing factors to the accident, but required training and certification has relied more on systems knowledge and individual demonstration of technical skills. This paper discusses some of the methods that have been used in an attempt to close the gap and improve the quality of aviation safety in the commercial airline field.

Commercial aviation in the 1960s showed a dramatic decline in the accident rates (Figure 1). This was due mostly to the improved reliability of jet turbine engines over reciprocating propeller technology. This period of time also witnessed the advent of advanced flight simulators which markedly reduced the number of aircraft accidents that occurred during training flights. Unfortunately, since that sharp decline in accident rates, the ratios have remained about constant. The public, however, looks at the total number of accidents, not at the ratios per 1,000 departures. With the booming increase in air travel, and the number of airlines and aircraft operating, the accident numbers will actually increase even though the system is becoming safer. This coupled with the increased size of commercial transports results in a situation where aviation safety and accident rates receive increased public scrutiny and government attention from the regulatory side.

All of this has placed inordinate pressure on the airline industry to improve safety in spite of an enviable record when compared with other forms of trans-

Figure 1. Accident Rates & Fatalities

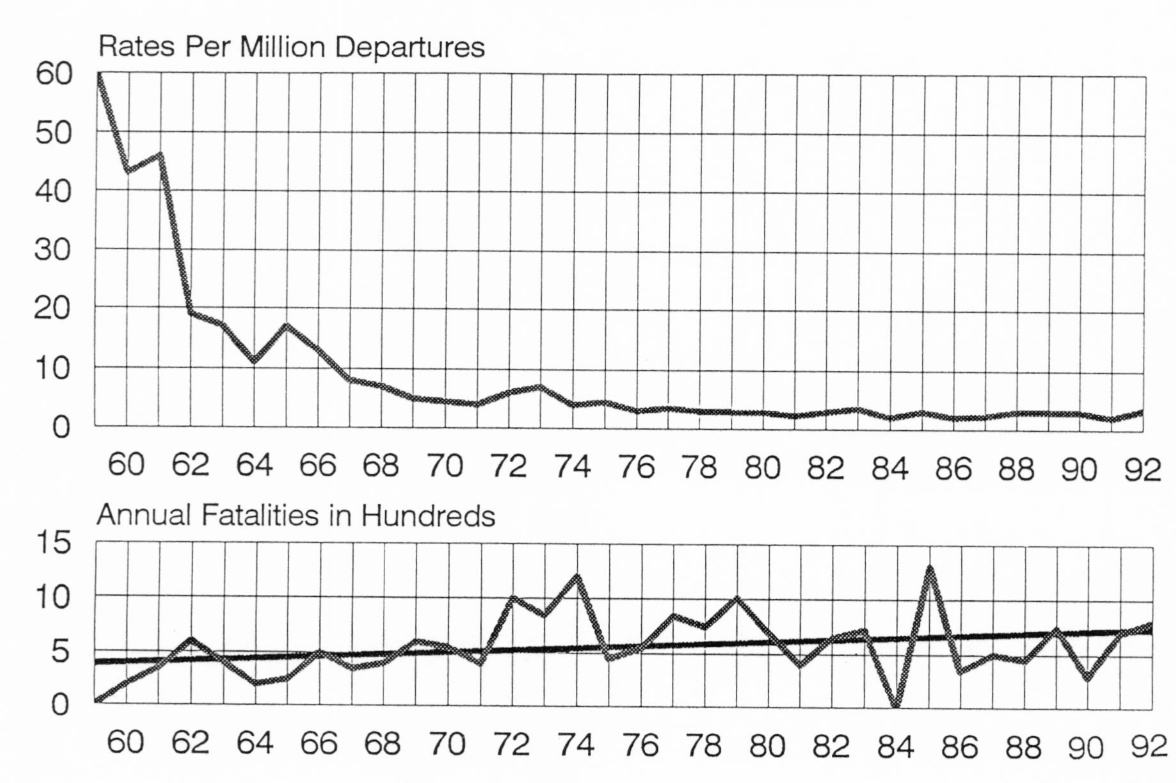

portation. In January of 1995, the FAA sponsored a major conference in Washington of all airline chief executive officers (CEOs) focused upon how to improve safety margins. Some airlines that have had a repetitive number of accidents over short periods of time have been singled out by the press, as well as regional carriers that train and certify their pilots to less stringent and demanding standards. At that conference, one particular training and certification method that has been in a test format for several years was singled out as being a contributor to improved safety. This program is labeled the AQP which stands for Advanced Qualification Program. This optional program is built on the following fundamentals:

1. Most aircraft accidents are due to a variety of factors including the involvement of the flight crew.
2. Most accidents are not due to individual pilot technical errors, but are due to problems of human interaction and crew problem-solving skills.[1]
3. Most traditional training and performance evaluation mandated and required by the FAA relies on individual technical maneuvers and individual technical skill performance.
4. The training and test situations are usually taken out of context from the actual operating environment. A pilot is presented with a particular technical problem such as the onset of an engine fire, and the pilot is then tested as to whether or not he/she can diagnose accurately the problem and follow the prescribed corrective procedure including using an appropriate checklist.

Historic attempts to improve safety records usually have included the acquisition and installation of more sophisticated engineering improvements to the airplane. These technology driven solutions have usually been coupled with increased levels of standardization and compliance surveillance by supervisors.

The FAA requires a commercial pilot to return to the airline's training center once or twice a year for a required proficiency check, and then on the alternate six months receive what is labeled as proficiency training. Every time the pilot comes into the training center his/her license is at stake. A recurring problem: What happens if an individual pilot does not pass a given set of technical maneuvers? In the event of a failure there, the pilot typically is recycled through the technical training system, given some additional training time in the simulator, and then receives another proficiency check (PC).

In comparison with aviation, other professional disciplines including medicine may have likewise concentrated on more sophisticated approaches to measuring technical competence of individuals operating in problem solving situations that are removed from the "Big Picture" of the real world.

Consequently, not only is the current aviation training system based on technical maneuvers and performance, but it is also binary in the sense of pass or fail. Perhaps one of the reasons why the existing system has remained the way it has for so long is that fact that collecting data on the basis of pass/fail does not yield very relevant data on how to improve the system itself. This coupled with a regulatory structure that moves at "glacial" speed has helped to prevent many innovations and new methods for training and establishing competency.

A case study of one airline's experience, United Airlines in the 1970s, is very informative. United suffered a string of hull loss accidents throughout the 70s which resulted in the destruction of several aircraft and loss of life. The final straw that precipitated management action was a Douglas DC-8 that crashed in Portland, Oregon in December of 1978. The aircraft had exhausted its fuel supply and crashed short of the airport. There was absolutely nothing wrong with the aircraft that would have prevented a safe conclusion to the flight. There was a mechanical problem when the landing gear was lowered and warning lights advising of a possible unsafe gear situation were illuminated. The crew worked through the appropriate checklists and prepared the cabin for an emergency landing, but still proceeded to circle and circle on an absolutely clear night until all fuel was used up. This was in spite of the fact that the flight engineer can be heard on the flight voice recorder advising the captain that fuel was running low. Although this accident had a mechanical problem as a trigger, it was crew coordination problems that ultimately led to the accident. The captain was considered an excellent pilot in the technical or "stick and rudder" sense and all pilots were trained in technical skills and systems knowledge.

This particular accident was the proverbial "last straw" for United Airlines. This crash and others led them to develop a human factors training and evaluation program to complement their existing technical training curriculum. All pilots were given specific training in human factors and teamwork skills, which was reinforced with simulator training. The simulator events were unique in the sense that an entire intact crew was provided with a mission scenario that was to be flown from beginning to end, with all the appropriate flight planning documents and other support material. The crew was presented with minor situations and technical problems along with other situations that required effective crew coordination for a successful resolution to the problem. United saw a dramatic change in their hull-loss safety record, and human factors training has been credited for a large part of their safety improvement experience.

Other airlines dismissed the United Airlines approach, and some were very vocal about not including human factors as part of their training curriculum. A common criticism heard was that the human factors part was too "touchy feely" or soft and could not be measured or evaluated in a concrete manner. Detractors would equate the United efforts as being akin to "charm school" or personality modification. This complaint has also been heard from some medical circles, and this argument was common in commercial airline aviation 10 years ago. Part of the reason is that technical trainers and check airmen (the supervisory pilots) are used to thinking in technical "stick-and-rudder" terms, such as plus or minus 100 feet, or "on glide-slope" or 10 knots fast. Their attitude is that these are areas that can be seen, observed and evaluated. They say "this is something I can see and rate. I can pass or fail a pilot on these terms." But terms such as leadership, assertion, situational awareness—these are seen as too remote from traditional technical training as well as soft and mushy issues. Consequently, the technical trainers and evaluators tended to avoid work in the human factors areas.

In 1987, Delta Airlines had a relatively unfortunate summer. Some may recall the David Letterman show which one evening featured the Delta Airlines Top Ten Marketing Slogans. The first one was "We never make the same mistake three times; a real man lands where he wants to; Delta is Amtrak with Wings." Delta had a Boeing 767 where the crew inadvertently turned off both engines shortly after takeoff from San Diego. The top ten slogan was "Noisy engines — we'll turn em off." Delta had a near miss with another aircraft over the North Atlantic. The slogan on Letterman was "Fly Delta where you can watch the in-flight movie on the aircraft next to you." Later Delta commented that all of these incidents and others were all rooted in human factors issues including communication, leadership, situational awareness, among others. The Delta attitude had been that the airline prided itself on its selection methods and only hired "captains." The airline focused on technical ability, technical training, and it was all centered on the individual as opposed to the crew.

With strong encouragement and counsel from the FAA, Delta began to implement a combination of training steps that were modeled after the work completed at United, Pan Am, and Alaska Airlines. These components further led to an industry working group that developed the training and certification standards for the Advanced Qualification Program (AQP) mentioned earlier. This new program is totally voluntary and optional, but is strongly recommended by the FAA and others. The components of the AQP are summarized in Figure 2, and they represent a sharp departure from the traditional training package.

1. The focus of training is the crew as well as the individual. This means that for a particular training cycle, a captain, and a first officer will train together along with a flight engineer (for specific aircraft). Traditional systems for training frequently paired two captains or two first officers together.
2. The training theme is crew-centered training including a human factors component along with technical training. It is important to recognize that evaluation of human factors issues cannot occur unless the crew has received specific training in this area.
3. The third focus area is Line Oriented Flight Training or LOFT As discussed earlier, the training in the simulator is based on an actual flight, in real time, with correct paper work. The instructor does not have the option of "freezing" the simulator and asking the crew what their intention is. Whatever the crew does, they live with, just as in the real world. Frequently, these LOFT scenarios are videotaped for later debriefing by the crew and their instructor. The tape is then erased.

4. The next element of the AQP process involves the collection and maintenance of data. The data is not collected on the binary pass/fail system, but is usually scaled data to represent various levels of passing, marginal performance, and unsatisfactory performance requiring rework or remediation. Data is collected over time, not for the purpose of looking at individual competency, but for the purpose of evaluating and analyzing the entire training and testing system. In this way, opportunities for improvement in training methods and focus areas can be diagnosed and implemented. In other areas, such as medicine, for data collection to be most useful requires that it be fed back to the training side of the organization. Even in aviation there is much room for improvement in categorizing the reasons for flight irregularities and other events so that the underlying causes of these situations can be identified.
5. The final focus is with evaluator skills. In aviation it was found that one of the major stumbling blocks was what items evaluators and testers focus upon. Many evaluators are uncomfortable with human factors issues primarily because they have never received training in this area. Another reason is that in some airlines human factors is an optional part of training. In the AQP system, it is a requirement and evaluators must receive specific training on how to recognize, assess, and debrief human factors issues.

The AQP experience is one that creates an opportunity for integrated training using a wider variety of class room and simulator experiences. Aviation has also learned that for human factors training to be successful, it must be operational and include a catalog of specific and observable crew behaviors. The industry is moving away from high-order words like judgment or leadership for example, because it is difficult to train evaluators reliably to assess these global terms. An example of something that is observable, concrete and assessable are the components of a crew briefing.[3] Pilots can be assessed on things they do or do not do such as—are the flight attendants briefed, are responsibilities for interfacing with automated systems covered, are expectations set for what a subordinate crew member is to do if non-standard procedures are observed. Specific behavioral markers are used which pilots can be trained to do, and which evaluators can be trained to observe with high reliability and agreement.

The experience in aviation has been that evaluation of human factors aspects is essential to improving performance in terms of system safety. Ten years ago the question that surfaced most often was whether or not human factors and crew resource management training actually worked and was beneficial. Today that question is no longer being debated.

It is still a struggle for many airlines to justify moving into this type of training and certification. It is an issue of cost and available time. While it is recognized that the AQP is definitely better training and certification due to the integration of technical and human factors aspects, it also requires more resources to implement and monitor. We also know that in aviation, there is rarely a single cause for an accident.[2] We will probably see the term "pilot error" used much less frequently as we gain more experience with identifying the various contributors to accidents and irregularities. Recent findings include accident contributors such as regulatory issues and organizational pressures. In more than a few accidents, the crew has been on duty for a high number of hours, they are getting a late start for the flight, there are delays in the system, there is pressure to hurry-up the process, and there may be a few factors at play such as weather or personal issues outside the routine flight factors. Consequently, in order to learn more about accident causes and solutions, the entire system requires examination.

Most of the major air carriers are in the process of implementing the AQP training and certification system. The process of integrating human factors and technical training is an ongoing effort for all the airlines involved and for the FAA as well. As evaluators become more skilled and as data collection efforts produce useful material, new training targets are identified. The increased use of automated aircraft with computerized flight management systems is demanding a whole new layer of training and testing. The training scenarios used in simulators are becoming more operational and challenging from the perspective of crew performance.

Airlines from around the world are beginning to adopt some of these methods, and this training is being extended beyond the cockpit door. Airlines are now doing interface training where pilots, flight attendants, dispatchers, gate agents, the FAA, and others involved with safety of flight operations receive specific training on crew coordination and problem solving. Issues of crew fatigue and steps that crew members can take to manage their own personal situations are now being covered in training, as well as the special training required for advanced technology flight decks.

The implications for medicine and other domains may be to learn from the aviation experience in transitioning from individual, technically centered training, to a system that zeroes in on crew performance in realistic settings where technical and human factors issues are integrated, not separated.

References

1. Cooper GE, White MD, Lauber JK. Resource management on the flight deck Moffett Field, CA: NASA-Ames Research Center, (*NASA Report No. CP2120*) 1979; 247 pp.247.

2. Helmreich RL. Human factors aspects of the Air Ontario crash at Dryden, Ontario: Analysis and recommendations. In V.P. Moshansky (Commissioner), *Commission of Inquiry into the Air Ontario Accident at Dryden, Ontario: Final Report. Technical Appendices,* 1992 Toronto, Ontario: Minister of Supply and Services, Canada; (pp. 319-348).

3. Helmreich RL, Butler RE, Taggart WR, Wilhelm JA. The NASA/University of Texas/FAA Line/LOS Checklist: A behavioral marker-based checklist for CRM skills assessment. *NASA/UT/FAA Technical Report 94-02* 1994, 4 pp.

CONCLUDING REMARKS

PART 8

Concluding Remarks

Gordon G. Page, Ed.D.
Keynote Speaker
University of British Columbia

Dr. Mancall: We asked Dr. Gordon Page to return for a few brief closing remarks to wind down the conference.

Dr. Page: Well, here we are at the end, and it's not possible to do justice to the richness of today's discussion in this last five minutes. The conference title, just to remind you, is *Assessing Clinical Reasoning: If Not the Oral Examination, What?* It's difficult and I would think incorrect to speak of the oral examination in the abstract. Each board, as we learned, uses the oral exam in very different ways. I will try to distill some common characteristics. First of all, the boards obviously devote a considerable amount of resources to this endeavor. They carefully train examiners; they standardize the examination across candidates; they monitor examiner consistency; and, they also monitor the quality of the examination most often through some form of statistical analysis.

Also discussed were some alternatives to the oral exam. These were: The key features problems, the computer-based simulations, and progress notes that are extracted in conjunction with standardized patient examinations. These are all viable options to consider when it comes to assessing reasoning-type skills in relation to physician performance.

I would like for a moment to recall last year's conference. Last year Christine McGuire, in her keynote address, suggested that a very clear definition of competence in each specialty should be prepared prior to developing assessment procedures. I would like to suggest that with this definition of competence in hand, the next logical step in developing board examinations is to select assessment procedures which most effectively assess various elements of competence. With respect to oral exams, the question therefore is not simply should they be used, but should they be used to assess defined aspects of competence.

I think it is a mistake to continue to label examinations by their format. We refer to multiple-choice examinations, oral examinations, computer examinations and so on. It may be more than a semantic difference if this notion were re-thought and examinations were labeled not by how they measure, but rather by what they measure. Such a change might permit a more productive and focused discussion on how to assess the various components of medical competence.

In closing, I recall being told that a definition of a good meeting is to acquire at least one good idea and meet one interesting person. Using this definition for a pass/fail criterion on this conference, I think that we would all agree that the conference was a huge success. Thank you.

Appendix I

Conference Participants

Faculty and Contributors

Philip G. Bashook, Ed.D.
Conference Coordinator
Director, Evaluation & Education
American Bd. Med. Specialties
1007 Church Street, Suite 404
Evanston, IL 60201

Isaac I. Bejar, Ph.D.
Principal Research Scientist
Educational Testing Service
Div. Cog. & Instruct. Science
Mail Stop 11 R
Princeton, NJ 08541

Robert W. Cantrell, M.D.
Executive Vice President
American Board of Otolaryngology
University of Virginia Med. Ctr.
Box 430 - Otolaryngology
Charlottesville, VA 22908

Brian E. Clauser, Ed.D.
National Board of Medical Examiners
3750 Market Street
Philadelphia, PA 19104-3190

Stephen G. Clyman, M.D.
Project Director, CBX
National Board Medical Examiners
3750 Market Street
Philadelphia, PA 19104-3190

W. Dale Dauphinee, M.D., FRCP(C)
Executive Director
Medical Council of Canada
Suite 300
2283 Boulevard St. Laurent
Ottawa, ON, Canada K1G 5A2

Jacques E. Des Marchais, M.D.
Vice Dean for Education
Université de Sherbrooke
Faculty of Medicine
3001 12th Avenue North
Sherbrooke, PQ, Canada, J1H 5N4

William Droegemueller, M.D.
UNC School of Medicine
Deptment Obstetrics/Gynecology, CB #7570
5007 Old Clinic Building
Chapel Hill, NC 27599-7570

Albert B. Gerbie, M.D.
Professor of Obstetrics/Gynecology
Northwestern University Med. School
707 N. Fairbanks Court, Suite 500
Chicago, IL 60611

Robert O. Guerin, Ph.D.
Vice President
American Board of Pediatrics
111 Silver Cedar Court
Chapel Hill, NC 27514-1651

Francis P. Hughes, Ph.D.
Executive Vice President
American Board of Anesthesiology
4101 Lake Boone Trail
The Summit Suite 510
Raleigh, NC 27607-7506

Mary E. Lunz, Ph.D.
Dir. Examination Activities
American Soc. Clin. Pathologists
Board of Registry
P.O. Box 12270
2100 West Harrison Street
Chicago, IL 60612-0270

Elliott L. Mancall, M.D.
Chairman, ABMS Committee on
Study of Eval. Proced. (COSEP)
Hahnemann University/Medical
College of Pennsylvania
Department of Neurology
Broad & Vine Streets
Philadelphia, PA 19102

Maurice J. Martin, M.D.
President, American Board of
Medical Specialties
Mayo Clinic, Department of Psychiatry
200 First Street, S.W.
Rochester, MN 55905

Donald E. Melnick, M.D.
Senior Vice President and
Vice President, Division
Evaluation Programs
National Board of Medical
Examiners
3750 Market Street
Philadelphia, PA 19104

Gordon G. Page, Ed.D.
Office of Coord., Health Sciences
University of British Columbia
Faculty of Medicine
#400, 2194 Health Sciences Mall
Vancouver, BC, Canada V6T 1Z3

Mary Ann Reinhart, Ph.D.
Associate Executive Director for
Evaluation and Research
American Board of Emergency
Medicine
3000 Coolidge Road
East Lansing, MI 48823

Stephen C. Scheiber, M.D.
Executive Vice President
American Board of Psychiatry &
Neurology
500 Lake Cook Road, Suite 335
Deerfield, IL 60015

Alfred E. Stillman, M.D.
Crozer Chester Medical Center
One Medical Center Boulevard
Upland, PA 19013

Paula L. Stillman, M.D.
Senior Associate Dean of
Postgraduate Education
Medical College of Pennsylvania/
Hahnemann University
Room 604 Quarters Building
3300 Henry Avenue
Philadelphia, PA 19129

William R. Taggart
Senior Research Associate
Aerospace Crew Research Project
NASA-Univ. of Texas-FAA
1609 Shoal Creek Blvd., #200
Austin, TX 78701

Youde Wang, Ph.D.
Education Specialist
Eastern Virginia Medical School
Office of Education
721 Fairfax Avenue
Norfolk, VA 23507

Conference Registrants

Herand Abcarian, M.D.
American Board Colon and
Rectal Surgery
20600 Eureka Road, Suite 713
Taylor, MI 48180

Maria Alonzi
American Board of Psychiatry
and Neurology
500 Lake Cook Road, Ste. 335
Deerfield, IL 60015

Edward R. Ames, D.V.M., Ph.D.
American Veterinary Medical Assn.
1931 N. Meacham Rd.
Shaumburg, IL 60173

William Ammons, D.D.S.
American Board of
Periodontology
720 Olive Way, Suite 610
Seattle, WA 98101

Rose Mary Ammons, Ed.D.
Professional Development
Technologies, Inc.
1440 Riverside Drive
Tarpon Springs, FL 34689

Irene Babcock
American Board of Colon
and Rectal Surgery
20600 Eureka Road, Suite 713
Taylor, MI 48180

Byron J. Bailey, M.D.
Treasurer, American Board of
Medical Specialties
University of Texas Medical Br.
Department of Otolaryngology
Room 7.104
John Sealy Hospital
Galveston, TX 77555-2704

H. Randolph Bailey, M.D.
6550 Fannin Street
Suite 2307
Houston, TX 77030-2723

David M. Barrett, M.D.
Mayo Clinic
200 First Street, SW
Rochester, MN 55905

Sorush Batmangelich, Ed.D.
BATM Medical Education
Consultants
3430 N. Lakeshore Dr., Ste. 8N
Chicago, IL 60657

John W. Becher, D.O.
American Osteopathic Board of
Emergency Medicine
One Lakeshore Drive
Newtown Square, PA 19073

John L. Bennett, M.Ed.
American Board of Podiatric Surgery
1601 Dolores Street
San Francisco, CA 94110-4906

Thomas W. Biester
American Board of Surgery
1617 John F. Kennedy Blvd, Suite 860
Philadelphia, PA 19103-1847

Jose Biller, M.D.
Indiana University School of Medicine
545 Barnhill Dr, Emerson Hall, Rm #125
Indianapolis, IN 46202-5124

Andre P. Boulais
Royal College of Physicians and Surgeons of Canada
774 Promenade Echo Drive
Ottawa, Ontario, Canada K1S 5N8

L. Thompson Bowles, M.D., Ph.D.
President
National Board of Medical Examiners
3750 Market Street
Philadelphia, PA 19104

John R. Boyce, D.V. M., Ph.D.
National Board Exam. Commission for Veterinary Medicine
1931 N. Meacham Road
Schaumburg, IL 60173-4360

Murray Brandstater, M.D.
Loma Linda University Medical Center
Dept. of Rehab Medicine, Rm A-237
11234 Anderson St
Loma Linda, CA 92354

Bertha L. Bullen, Ph.D.
American Board of Emergency Medicine
3000 Coolidge Road
East Lansing, MI 48823

Jane V. Bunce
American Board of Surgery
1617 John F. Kennedy Blvd, Ste 860
Philadelphia, PA 19103-1847

Albert E. Burns, D.P.M.
American Board of Podiatric Surgery
669 Crespi Drive, #B
Pacifica, CA 94044-3430

Tom Campbell, M.D.
American Association of Physician Specialists
P.O. Box 100
Bradford, TN 38316

M. Paul Capp, M.D.
American Board of Radiology
5255 E. Williams Circle, Suite 6800
Tucson, AZ 85711

Jan A. Carline, Ph.D.
University of Washington School of Medicine
1959 NE Pacific St, RH-20
Seattle, WA 98195

Joseph E. Clinton, M.D.
Hennepin County Medical Center
Department of Emergency Medicine
701 Park Avenue
Minneapolis, MN 55415

William Coke, M.D., FRCPC
C/O Department of Medical Health Science Center
GC410-820 Sherbrook Street
Winnipeg, Manitoba
Canada R3A 1R9

George E. Cruft, M.D.
American Board of Surgery
1617 John F. Kennedy Blvd., Suite 860
Philadelphia, PA 19103-1847

Bruce F. Cullen, M.D.
Harbor View Medical Center
325 9th Avenue
Seattle, WA 98104

Anita Curran, M.D., M.P.H.
UMDNJ Robert Wood Johnson
Medical School
1 Robert Wood Johnson Place
MEB Bldg, Rm 204
New Brunswick, NJ 08903

Joel A. DeLisa, M.D.
UMDNJ New Jersey Medical School
150 Bergen St., University Heights
Newark, NJ 17103-2406

David R. DeMarais
American Dental Association
211 E. Chicago Avenue
Chicago, IL 60611

Harold M. Dick, M.D.
Columbia-Presbyterian Med Ctr
622 W. 168 St., #PH5-129
New York, NY 10032

Charles W. Dohner, Ph.D.
University of Washington School
of Medicine
Department of Medical Educ
E312 Hlth Sci Bldg., SC45
Seattle, WA 98195

Sandra Dolan, Ph.D.
American Osteopathic Association
142 E. Ontario
Chicago, IL 60611

Stewart B. Dunsker, M.D.
Mayfield Neurological Institute
2123 Auburn Avenue, Suite 431
Cincinnati, OH 45219

Cindy Durley
Dental Assisting National Board
216 E. Ontario Street
Chicago, IL 60611

Mark L. Dyken, M.D.
Indiana University
School of Medicine
Department of Neurology
1001 W Tenth St., Ste. B-402
Indianapolis, IN 46202

Gerald Felsenthal, M.D.
Sinai Hospital of Baltimore
2401 W. Belvedere Avenue
Baltimore, MD 21215

Benjamin A. Field, D.O., ACOEP
American Osteopathic Board of
Emergency Medicine
4207 E. Vogel Avenue
Phoenix, AZ 85028

Gregory S. Fortna
American Board of Psychiatry and
Neurology
500 Lake Cook Road, Ste. 335
Deerfield, IL 60015

Katherine V. Gabbard
American Podiatric Med Spec Bd
15595 East Street
Marcellus, MI 49067

Alberto Galofre, M.D.
St. Louis University
School of Medicine
1402 S. Grand Blvd.
St. Louis, MO 63104

Bruce M. Gans, M.D.
Rehabilitation Institute of Michigan
261 Mack Boulevard
Detroit, MI 48201

Craig Gjerde, Ph.D.
University of Wisconsin-Madison
1300 University Ave., 2020 MSC
Madison, WI 53706

Gerald S. Golden, M.D.
National Board of Medical Examiners
3750 Market Street
Philadelphia, PA 19104

Greg Gormanous, Ph.D.
Association of State & Provincial Psychology Boards
Louisiana State University-Alexandria
8100 Highway 71 South
Alexandria, LA 71302-91921

George Gray, Ed.D.
American College Testing
2201 N. Dodge
Iowa City, IA 52243

Leon Gross, Ph.D.
National Board of Examiners in Optometry
4340 East West Highway, Suite 1010
Bethesda, MD 20814

Charles L. Haine, O.D.
National Board of Examiners in Optometry
4340 East West Highway
Bethesda, MD 20814

Kerry Hamsher, Ph.D.
American Board of Clinical Neuropsychology
1218 W. Kilbourn Ave., Ste. 415
Milwaukee, WI 53233-1325

Norman R. Hertz, Ph.D.
California State Department of Consumer Affairs
400 R Street, Suite 1070
Sacramento, CA 95814

Kaaren I. Hoffman, Ph.D.
University of Southern California School of Medicine
Division of Research
1975 Zonal Avenue, KAM-200
Los Angeles, CA 90033-1039

Joseph C. Honet, M.D.
Sinai Hospital of Detroit
6767 W. Outer Drive
Detroit, MI 48235

Harry J. Hurley, M.D.
American Board of Dermatology
Henry Ford Hospital
1 Ford Place
Detroit, MI 48202-3450

Fred M. Jacobs, M.D., J.D.
New Jersey State Board of Medical Examiners
Saint Barnabas Medical Center
Old Short Hills Road
Livingston, NJ 07039

Cathy Johnson
Applied Measurement Professionals
8310 Nieman Road
Lenexa, KS 66214

Dorthea Juul, Ph.D.
American Board of Psychiatry and Neurology
500 Lake Cook Road, Ste. 335
Deerfield, Il 60015

George W. Kaplan, M.D.
Pediatric Urology Association
7930 Frost St., Suite 407
San Diego, CA 92123

John P.W. Kelly, D.M.D, M.D.
American Board of Oral & Maxillofacial Surgery
625 N. Michigan Avenue
Chicago, IL 60611

Jack D. Kerth, M.D.
303 E. Chicago Avenue
Chicago, IL 60611

William Killoy, D.D.S.
University of Missouri Kansas School of Dentistry
650 East 25th Street
Kansas City, MO 64108

Mary M. Kino, Ph.D.
The Psychological Corporation
555 Academic Court
San Antonio, TX 78204

Lenora G. Knapp, Ph.D.
Knapp & Associates
217 S. Harrison St
Princeton, NJ 08540

Allan E. Kolker, M.D.
Washington University School of Medicine
660 South Euclid Avenue
St. Louis, MO 63110

Bernard M. Lefebvre, M.D.
Royal College of Physicians and Surgeons of Canada
774 Promenade Echo Drive
Ottawa, Ontario
Canada K1S 5N8

Edward A. Lichter, M.D.
University of Illinois at Chicago College of Medicine
840 South Wood Street
Chicago, IL 60612-7323

Steven A. Lieberman, M.D.
University of Texas Medical Branch
301 University Blvd., MRB 3.142
Galveston, TX 77555-1060

John H. Littlefield, Ph.D.
Office of Educational Resources
University of Texas Health Science Center
7703 Floyd Curl Drive
San Antonio, Texas 78284-7896

Glennis G. Lundberg
American Board of Thoracic Surgery
One Rotary Center, Suite 803
Evanston, IL 60201

Sandra Madison, D.D.S., M.S.
American Board of Endodontics
5 Yorkshire St., Suite B
Asheville, NC 28803

Charlene Martin
American Board of Periodontology
University of Maryland, Baltimore College of Dental Surgery
666 W. Baltimore St., Room 3-C-08
Baltimore, MD 21201

Denise Massey
Royal College of Physicians and Surgeons of Canada
774 Promenade Echo Dr.
Ottawa, Ontario
Canada K1S 5N8

M. Jane Matjasko, M.D.
University of Maryland
Medical System
22 South Greene St., Suite 511C
Baltimore, MD 21201

William C. McGaghie, Ph.D.
Northwestern University
Medical School
303 East Chicago, 3-13
Chicago, IL 60611

Donald E. Melnick, M.D.
National Board of Medical
Examiners
3750 Market Street
Philadelphia, PA 19104

Thomas C. Meyer, M.D.
University of Wisconsin
2715 Marshall Ct.
Madison, WI 53705

John D. Milam, M.D.
UTHSC-H Medical School
Pathology and Laboratory
Medicine
P.O. Box 20708
Houston, TX 77225

Benson S. Munger, Ph.D.
American Board of
Emergency Medicine
3000 Coolidge Road
East Lansing, MI 48879

Stan Niemiec
American Board of
Psychiatry and Neurology
500 Lake Cook Rd., Suite 335
Deerfield, IL 60015

Patricia J. Numann, M.D.
American Board of Surgery
Department of Surgery
SUNY Health Science Center
at Syracuse
750 East Adams Street
Syracuse, NY 13210

Ronald J. Nungester, Ph.D.
National Board of Medical
Examiners
3750 Market Street
Philadelphia, PA 19104

Mary J. O'Sullivan, M.D.
Department of Obstetrics and
Gynecology
University of Miami
1611 NW 12th Ave.,
East Tower, Rm. 4070
Miami, FL 33136

Burton M. Onofrio, M.D.
Mayo Clinic
Department of Neurosurgery
200 First St, SW
Rochester, NM 55905

Joachim L. Opitz, M.D.
American Board of Physical
Medicine and Rehabilitation
Norwest Center, Ste. 674
21 First St, SW
Rochester, MN 55902

William D. Owens, M.D.
Washington University School of
Medicine
Department of Anesthesiology
660 South Euclid Avenue
St. Louis, MO 63110

Louise Papineau
Royal College of Physicians and Surgeons of Canada
774 Promenade Echo Drive
Ottawa, Ontario
Canada K1S 5N8

Robert Pascuzzi, M.D.
Indiana University
Department of Neurology, Regenstrief Center, 6th Floor
1050 Walnut Street
Indianapolis, IN 46077

Israel Penn, M.D.
University of Cincinnati
231 Bethesda Ave, ML 0558
Cincinnati, OH 45267-0558

Floyd Pennington, Ph.D.
American Association of Physician Specialists
804 Main St, Suite D
Forest Park, GA 30050

Alan D. Perlmutter, M.D.
American Board of Urology
31700 Telegraph Rd., Suite 150
Bingham Farms, MI 48025

Oleg Petrov, D.P.M.
American Board of Podiatric Orthopaedic and Primary Podiatric Medicine
111 N. Wabash Ave, Suite 1914
Chicago, IL 60602

George Podgorny, M.D.
Bowman Gray School of Medicine
2115 Georgia Avenue
Winston-Salem, NC 27104

Martin M. Pressman, D.P.M.
American Board of Podiatric Surgery
32 Cherry Street
Milford, CT 06460-3413

Paul R. Quintavalle, D.P.M.
American Board of Podiatric Surgery
879 Haddon Avenue
Collingswood, NJ 08108-1941

Michael M. Ravitch, Ph.D.
Northwestern University Medical School
303 E. Chicago Avenue, 3-13
Chicago, IL 60611

Christine Reidy
Commission on Dietetic Registration
216 W. Jackson Boulevard
Chicago, IL 60606-6995

Alice R. Ring, M.D., M.P.H.
American Board of Preventive Medicine
9950 W. Lawrence Ave., Suite 106
Schiller Park, IL 60176

Stanley D. Roberts, M.B., Ch.B.
The Royal College of Physicians of Ireland
6 Kildare Street
Dublin 2, Ireland

Gerald A. Rosen, Ph.D.
Sylvan Technology Centers
3435 Central Avenue
Huntingdon Valley, PA 19006

David A. Rothenberger, M.D.
2550 University Avenue, W, #313N
St. Paul, MN 55114-1084

Deborah C. Rugg, Ph.D.
Carle Foundation Hospital
611 W. Park
Urbana, IL 61801

Pedro Ruiz, M.D.
University of Texas Medical School at Houston
Mental Sciences Institute
1300 Moursund St
Houston, TX 77030

Joseph F. Sackett, M.D.
University of Wisconsin Hospital and Clinic
Department of Radiology
600 Highland Avenue
Madison, WI 53792-3252

Lawrence Saidman, M.D.
University of California, San Diego
Medical Center (UCSD)
9500 Gilman Drive
La Jolla, CA 92093-0815

Burton Sandok, M.D.
Mayo Medical School
200 First St, SW
Rochester, MN 55905

Edward J. Sarama, D.O.
American Osteopathic Board of Emergency Medicine
142 E. Ontario
Chicago, IL 60611

Richard Sarles, M.D.
Division of Child and Adolescent Psychology
University of Maryland
645 West Redwood St.
Baltimore, MD 21201

David J. Schoetz, Jr., M.D.
Lahey Clinic
41 Mall Road
Burlington, MA 01805

Lois L. Schuhrke
American Dental Association
211 E. Chicago Avenue
Chicago, IL 60643

Joyce Sigmon
American Academy of Implant Dentistry
211 East Chicago Avenue
Chicago, IL 60611

Michael Simon, M.D.
University of Chicago
5841 S. Maryland, MC3079
Chicago, IL 60637

Fred G. Smith, M.D.
American Board of Pediatrics
111 Silver Cedar Court
Chapel Hill, NC 27514

Joseph F. Smoley, Ph.D.
National Board of Osteopathic Medicine Examiners
2700 River Rd., Suite #407
Des Plaines, IL 60018

Steven M. Spinner, D.P.M.
American Board of Podiatric Surgery
301 N.W. 84th Avenue
Plantation, FL 33324-1852

Robert S. Staffanou, D.D.S.
American Board of Prosthodontics
1930 Sea Way
P.O. Box 1409
Bodega Bay, CA 94923-1409

Christopher L. Surek, D.O.
Resurrection Medical Center
7447 West Talcott
Chicago, IL 60631

Jacques L. Surer, Jr., D.O.
American Osteopathic Board of Ophthalmology and Otolaryngology
1750 5th Avenue
York, PA 17403

Alton I. Sutnick, M.D.
Educational Commission for Foreign Medical Graduates
3624 Market Street
Philadelphia, PA 19104

Roy A. Swift, Ph.D., OTR
American Occupational Therapy Certification Board
4 Research Place
Rockville, MD 20850

Susan Swing
Accreditation Council for Graduate Medical Education
515 N. State St
Chicago, IL 60610

Peter E. Tanguay, M.D.
Bingham Child Guidance Clinic
200 East Chestnut St
Louisville, KY 40292

Stephen J. Thomas, M.D.
New York Hospital-Cornell University Medical Center (NYH-CUMC)
525 E. 68th Street
New York, NY 10021

Frank L. Thorne, M.D.
1229 Madison
Seattle, WA 98104

William F. Todd, D.P.M.
American Board of Podiatric Surgery
21230 Dequindre Road
Warren, MI 48091-2279

Margaret F. Traband, M.Ed., R.R.T.
University of Toledo
2600 Nebraska
Toledo, OH 43606

Michael J. Trepal, D.P.M.
American Board of Podiatric Surgery
115 Henry Street
Brooklyn, NY 11201-2562

Nicholas Vick, M.D.
Evanston Hospital
2650 Ridge Avenue
Evanston, IL 60201

Dale Wade, D.D.S.
American Board of Orthodontics
3220 Riverside Dr.
Columbus, OH 43221

Nicolas E. Walsh, M.D.
UTHSC - San Antonio
7703 Floyd Curl Drive
San Antonio, TX 78287-7798

Victor W. Waymouth, B.Ed., M.D.
College of Physicians and Surgeons of British Columbia
1807 West 10th Avenue
Vancouver, B.C., Canada V3J 3T8

Lynn C. Webb, Ed.D.
National Board of Medical Examiners
3750 Market Street
Philadelphia, PA 19104

Cynthia Welsh
Educational Testing Service
Rosedale Road (37P)
Princeton, NJ 08541

Gerald P. Whelan, M.D.
American Board of Emergency Medicine
3000 Coolidge Road
East Lansing, MI 48823-6319

Loretta F. Wilkinson, Ph.D.
Northeastern Ohio Universities College of Medicine
4209 State Route 44, PO Box 95
Rootstown, OH 44272

Caryn Wilson
American Board of Otolaryngology
5615 Kirby Drive, Suite 936
Houston, TX 77005

James M. Woolfenden, M.D.
Arizona Health Science Center
Division of Nuclear Medicine
1501 N. Campbell
Tucson, AZ 85724

James E. Youker, M.D.
Medical College of Wisconsin
C/O Doyne Clinic
8700 W. Wisconsin Avenue
Milwaukee, WI 53226

Committee on Study of Evaluation Procedures (COSEP)

***Elliott L. Mancall, M.D.**
Hahnemann University–Medical College of Pennsylvania
Department of Neurology
Broad & Vine Streets
Philadelphia, PA 19102

George E. Cruft, M.D.
American Board of Surgery
1617 John F. Kennedy Blvd.
Suite 860
Philadelphia, PA 19103-1847

Joel A. DeLisa, M.D.
UMDNJ Medical School, University Heights
University Hospital, Room B-261
150 Bergen Street
Newark, NJ 07103-2406

Stewart B. Dunsker, M.D
Mayfield Neurological Institute
2123 Auburn Avenue, Suite 431
Cincinnati, OH 45219

***Francis P. Hughes, Ph.D.**
American Board of Anesthesiology
100 Constitution Plaza
Hartford, CT 06103-1796

Edward A. Krull, M.D.
Department of Dermatology
Henry Ford Hospital
Detroit, MI 48202

Charles L. Puckett, M.D.
University of Missouri Medical Center M-349
One Hospital Drive
Columbia, MO 65201-5276

***Mary Ann Reinhart, Ph.D.**
American Board of Emergency Medicine
3000 Coolidge Road
East Lansing, MI 48823

Fred G. Smith, M.D.
American Board of Pediatrics
111 Silver Cedar Court
Chapel Hill, NC 27514-1651

*Conference Planning Committee

Conference Staff

Maxima Avila
*Philip G. Bashook, Ed.D.
Marci Burr
J. Lee Dockery, M.D.
Bobbye Higdon
Kathleen Hoinacki
Evalyn Moore
Alexis Rodgers
Gail Strejc
Kathy Szarnych

Appendix II

Bibliography

1. Abrahamson S. The oral examination: The case for and the case against. In Lloyd JS; Langsley DG (Eds.): *Evaluating the Skills of Medical Specialists.* Evanston, IL: American Board of Medical Specialties; 1983 pp. 121-124.

2. Advisory Board for Medical Specialties. Round Table Conference, The evaluation of the qualifications of candidates for certification by American Boards in the specialties (pp. 24-80), *Proceedings*, February 5, 1950 (Mimeograph).

3. Alexander PA; Kulikowich JM; Jetton TL. The role of subject-matter knowledge and interest in the processing of linear and nonlinear texts. *Rev Educ Res*; 1994;64:201-252.

4. American Board of Pediatric Dentistry Clinical Section: Case Review Option. *Pediatr Dentistry*; 1993;15:53-64.

5. Anbar M. Comparing assessments of students' knowledge by computerized open-ended and multiple-choice tests. *Acad Med*; 1991;66:420-422.

6. Anderson EG. The "special competency" exam revisited - and rebuked. *Geriatrics*; 1990;45:75-76.

7. Arndt CB; Guly UMV; McManus IC. Preclinical anxiety: The stress associated with a viva voce examination. *Med Educ*; 1986;20:274-280.

8. Arrow H; McGrath JE. Membership matters: How member change and continuity affect small group structure, process, and performance. *Small Group Res*; 1993;24:334-361.

9. Barnes EJ; Pressy DL. The reliability and validity of oral examinations. *School and Society*; 1929;30:719-722.

10. Bashook PG. Beyond the traditional written and oral examinations: New certification methods. In Shore JH; Scheiber SC (Eds.): *Certification, Recertification, and Lifetime Learning in Psychiatry.* Washington, DC: Am Psychiatr Press, Inc; 1994, pp. 117-138.

11. Bauer MI; Johnson-Laird P. How diagrams can improve reasoning. *Psychol Sci*; 1993; 4:372-378.

12. Beaulieu MD; Leclere H; Bordage G. Taxonomy of difficulties in general practice. *Can Fam Phys*; 1993;39:1369-1375.

13. Beaumier A; Bordage G; Saucier D; Turgeon J. Nature of the clinical difficulties of first-year family residents under direct observation. *Can Med Assoc J*; 1992;146:489-497.

14. Bejar II; Braun HI. On the synergy between assessment and instruction: Early lessons from computer-based simulations. *Machine-Mediated Learning*; 1994;4:5-25.

15. Berk SL; Harvill LM; Douglas JE. A senior oral examination to test clinical skills developed during a subinternship. *Teach Learn Med*; 1989;1:97-100.

16. Blumenthal D. Making medical errors in "Medical treasures." *JAMA* 1994;272:1867-1868.

17. Bonfiglio M. Experiments in revision of the oral examination: American Orthopaedic Surgery. In Lloyd JS; Langsley DG (Eds.): *Evaluating the Skills of Medical Specialists.* American Board of Medical Specialties, Evanston, IL; 1983, pp. 125-128.

18. Bordage G. Elaborated knowledge: A key to successful diagnostic thinking. *Acad Med*; 1994;69:883-885.

19. Bordage G; Brailovsky C; Carretier H; Page G. Content validation of key features on a national examination of clinical decision-making skills. *Acad Med;* 1995;70:276-281.

20. Bordage G; Lemieux M. Semantic structures and diagnostic thinking of experts and novices. *Acad Med*; 1991;66:S70-S72.

21. Bordage G; Grant J; Marsden P. Quantitative assessment of diagnostic ability. *Med Educ*; 1990;24:413-425.

22. Bordage G; Lemieux M. Some cognitive characteristics of medical students with and without diagnostic reasoning difficulties. *Proceedings,* Ann Conf Res Med Educ, Assoc Am Med Coll; 1986;25:185-190.

23. Bordage G.; Zacks R. The structure of medical knowledge in the memories of medical students and general practitioners: Categories and prototypes. *Med Educ*; 1984;18:406-416.

24. Bordage G.; Page G. An alternative approach to PMPs: The key features' concept. In Hart I & Harden R (Eds.): *Further Developments in Assessing Clinical Competence* (pp. 59-75). Montreal, Quebec: *Can-Heal Publ*; 1987.

25. Bowles LT. A worthy search: The development of the key-features concept. *Acad Med*; 1995;70:89-90.

26. Brailovsky CA; Bordage G; Allen T; Dumont H. Writing vs. coding diagnostic impressions in an examination: Short-answer vs. long-menu responses. *Proceedings,* Ann Conf Res Med Educ, Assoc Am Med Coll; 1988;27:201-206.

27. Bridgeman B; Rock DA. Relationships among multiple-choice and open-ended analytical questions. *J Educ Meas*; 1993;30:313-329.

28. Butzin DW; Finberg L; Brownlee RC; Guerin, RO. Study of the reliability of the grading process used in the American Board of Pediatrics' oral examination. *J Med Educ*; 1982; 57:944-946.

29. Calfee R. Paper, pencil, potential, and performance. *Curr Dir Psychol Sci*; 1993;2:6-7.

30. Carter HD. How reliable are good oral examinations? *Calif J Educ Res*; 1962;13:147-153.

31. Case SM; Swanson DB; Woolliscroft JO. Assessment of diagnostic pattern recognition skills in medicine clerkships using a written test. In Harden RM; Hart IR; Mulholland H (Eds.) *International Conference Proceedings*: Approaches to the assessment of clinical competence. Part 2. Dundee, Scottish Centre for Medical Education; 1992, pp. 452-458.

32. Ceci S; Liker J. Academic and nonacademic intelligence: An experimental separation. In Sternberg RF & Wagner RK (Eds.): *Practical Intelligence.* New York: Cambridge Univ Press; 1986, pp. 119-142.

33. Clauser BE; Clyman SG. A contrasting groups' approach to standard setting for performance assessments of clinical skills. *Acad Med*; 1994;69:S42-S44.

34. Clauser BE; Ross LP; Clyman SG; Rose KM; Margolis MJ; Nungester RJ. Development of a scoring algorithm to replace expert rating for scoring a complex performance-based assessment. Ann Meeting Nat Council Measurement Educ, San Francisco, CA, April 18-22, 1995. (Unpublished manuscript).

35. Clyman SG; Melnick DE; Julian ER; Orr NA; Cotton KE. *The National Board of Medical Examiners' computer-based examination clinical simulation (CBX).* Philadelphia, PA: National Board of Medical Examiners, 1991, pp. 1-51. (Monograph)

36. Colton T; Peterson OL. An assay of medical students' abilities by oral examination. *J Med Educ*; 1967;42:1005-1014.

37. Cox K. How to improve oral examinations. *Med J Aust*; 1978;2:476-477.

38. Cox J; Mulholland H. An instrument for assessment of videotapes of general practitioners' performance. *Br Med J*; 1993;306:1043-1046.

39. Dauphinee D; Case S; Fabb W; McAvoy P; Saunders N; Wakeford R. Standard setting for recertification. In Newble D; Jolly B; Wakeford R (Eds.): *The Certification and Recertification of Doctors: Issues in the Assessment of Clinical Competence.* Great Britain: Cambridge Univ Press; 1994, pp. 201-215.

40. Dauphinee WD; Prosser RJ; Rothman AI; McLean LD. Improving oral examinations: The usefulness of statistical analysis. In Hart IR; Harden RM; Des Marchais J (Eds.) *International Conference Proceedings*: Current Developments in Assessing Clinical Competence. Montreal, Quebec: Can-Heal Publ, Inc; 1992, 285-288.

41. Day SC; Norcini JJ; Diserens D; Cebul RD; Schwartz S; Beck LH; Webster GD; Schnabel, TG; Elstein, A. The validity of an essay test of clinical judgment. *Acad Med*; 1990;65:S39-S40.

42. Eagle CJ; Martineau R; Hamilton K. The oral examination in anaesthetic resident evaluation. *Can J Anaesth*; 1993;40:947-53.

43. Easton R. Differences between oral examination grades given by doctor-nurse pairs. *Br J Med Educ;* 1968;2:301-302.

44. Elstein AS; Shulman LS; Sprafka SA. *Medical Problem Solving: An Analysis of Clinical Reasoning.* Cambridge, MA: Harvard Univ Press; 1978, pp. 1-323.

45. Evans LR; Ingersoll RW; Smith EJ. The reliability, validity, and taxonomic structure of the oral examination. *J Med Educ*; 1966;41:651-657.

46. Foster JT; Abrahamson S; Lass S; Girard R; Garris R. Analysis of an oral examination used in specialty board certification. *J Med Educ*; 1969;44:951-954.

47. Foukles J; Bandaranayake R; Hays R; Phillips G; Rothman A; Southgate L; Wakeford R. Combining components of assessment. In Newble D; Jolly B; Wakeford, R (Eds.) *International Conference Proceedings*: The certification and recertification of doctors: Issues in the assessment of clinical competence. Great Britain: Cambridge Univ Press; 1994, pp. 134-150.

48. Gigone D; Hastie R. The common knowledge effect: Information sharing and group judgment. *J Pers Soc Psychol*; 1993;65:959-974.

49. Ginsburg AD. Comparison of intraining evaluation with tests of clinical ability in medical students. *J Med Educ*; 1985;60:29-36.

50. Grand'Maison P; Lescop J; Rainsberry P; Brailovsky, CA. Large-scale use of an objective, structured clinical examination for licensing family physicians. *Can Med Assoc J*; 1992;146:1735-1740.

51. Green E; Evans LR; Ingersoll RW. The reactions of students in the oral examination. *J Med Educ*; 1967;42:345-349.

52. Halio JL. Ph.D.'s and the oral examination. *J Higher Educ*; 1963;34:148-152.

53. Holloway PJ; Collins CK; Start KB. Reliability of viva voce examinations. *Br Dent J*; 1968;125:211-214.

54. Holloway PJ; Hardwick JL; Morris J; Start KB. The validity of essays and viva voca examining techniques. *Br Dent J*; 1967;123:227-232.

55. Hout B. Reliability, validity, and holistic scoring: What we know and what we need to know. *Coll Compos & Comm*; 1990;41:201-213.

56. Huang RR; Maatsch J; Downing S; Douglas B; Munger B. Reliability and validity of ratings of physician performance. *Proceedings,* Ann Conf Res Med Educ, Assoc Am Med Coll; November 1984: 70-75.

57. Hubbard JP; Levitt EJ; Schumacher CF; Schnabel TG. An objective evaluation of clinical competence. *N Engl J Med*; 1965;272:1321-1328.

58. Jacques A; Sindon A; Bourque A; Bordage G; Ferland, JJ. A structured oral interview for the identification of educational needs of family physicians: Development and pilot test. *Can Fam Phys*, 1995 (In press).

59. Jain SS; DeLisa JA; Campagnolo DI. Methods used in the evaluation of clinical competency of physical medicine and rehabilitation residents. *Am J Phys Med Rehabil*; 1994;73:234-239.

60. Jensen AR. Test validity: g versus "Tacit knowledge." *Curr Dir Psychol Sci*; 1993;2:9-10.

61. Juul D; Scheiber SC. The part II psychiatry examination: Facts about the oral examination. In Shore JH; Scheiber SC (Eds.): *Certification, Recertification, and Lifetime Learning in Psychiatry.* Washington, DC: Am Psychiatr Press, Inc; 1994, pp. 71-90.

62. Kane M. Validating the performance standards associated with passing scores. *Rev Educ Res*; 1994;64:425-461.

63. Kassebaum DG; Szenas PL. The longer road to medical school graduation. *Acad Med*; 1994;69:856-860.

64. Katz PP; Costantino CM; Hengl, RD. *Certified dental assistant examination validation.* Chicago, IL: Dental Assisting National Board, Inc; 1994, pp. 1-49. (Project Report)

65. Kelley PR; Matthews JH; Schumacher CF. Analysis of oral examination of the American Board of Anesthesiology. *J Med Educ*; 1971;46:982-988.

66. Kittle CF. Experiments in revision of the oral examination: American Board of Thoracic Surgery (The examination of a young surgeon). In Lloyd JS; Langsley DG (Eds): *Evaluating the Skills of Medical Specialists.* Evanston, IL: American Board of Medical Specialties; 1983, pp. 105-109.

67. Kline SA; Fleming SA. Passing the oral examination for specialist qualification in Psychiatry: Part II. *Can J Psychiatry*; 1989;34:925-926.

68. Leape LL. Error in medicine. *JAMA*; 1994;272:1851-1857.

69. Leclere H; Beaulieu MD; Bordage G; Sindon A; Couillard M. Why are clinical problems difficult? General practitioners' opinions concerning 24 clinical problems. *Can Med Assoc J*; 1990;143:1305-1315.

70. Leichner P; Sisler GC; Harper D. The clinical oral examination in psychiatry: Association between subscoring and global marks. *Can J Psychiatry*; 1986; 31:750-751.

71. Levine HG; McGuire CH. The use of role-playing to evaluate affective skills in medicine. *J Med Educ*; 1970(b);45:700-705.

72. Levine HG; McGuire CH. The validity and reliability of oral examinations in assessing cognitive skills in medicine. *J Educ Meas*; 1970(a);7:63-73.

73. Lindsay JF. Studies of the oral examination: The examination in pediatric cardiology. In Lloyd JS; Langsley DG (Eds.): *Evaluating the Skills of Medical Specialists.* Evanston, IL: American Board of Medical Specialties; 1983, pp. 111-114.

74. Lipscomb PR. Summary of conference on oral examinations. In Lloyd JS; Langsley DG (Eds.): *Evaluating the Skills of Medical Specialists.* Evanston, IL: American Board of Medical Specialties; 1983, pp. 137-140.

75. Ludbrook JH; Marshall VR. Examiner training for clinical examinations. *Brit J Med Educ*; 1971;5:152-155.

76. Lukhele R; Thissen D; Wainer H. On the relative value of multiple-choice, constructed response, and examinee-selected items on two achievement tests. *J Educ Meas*; 1994;31:234-250.

77. Lunz ME; Bergstrom BA. An empirical study of computerized adaptive test administration conditions. *J Educ Meas*; 1994;31:251-263.

78. Lunz ME; Stahl JA. The effect of rater severity on person ability measure: A Rasch model analysis. *Am J Occup Ther*; 1993;47:311-317.

79. Lunz ME; Stahl JA. Judge consistency and severity across grading periods. *Eval Hlth Prof*; 1990;13:425-444.

80. Lunz ME; Stahl JA; Wright BD. Interjudge reliability and decision reproducibility. *Educ Psychol Meas*; 1994;54:913-925.

81. Lunz ME; Stahl JA. Impact of examiners on candidate scores: An introduction to the use of multifacet Rasch Model Analysis for oral examinations. *Teach Learn Med*; 1993;5:174-181.

82. Maatsch JL; Munger BS; Podgorny G. On the reliability and validity of the board examination in Emergency Medicine. In Wolcott B; Rund D (Eds.): *Emergency Medicine Annual.* Norwalk, CT: Appleton-Century-Crofts; 1982, pp. 183-222.

83. Maatsch JL; Huang RR; Downing S; Barker D; Munger B. The predictive validity of test formats and a psychometric theory of clinical competence. *Proceedings,* Ann Conf Res Med Educ, Assoc Am Med Coll; November 1984: 76-82.

84. Magarian GJ; Mazur DJ. Evaluation of students in medicine clerkships. *Acad Med*; 1990;65:341-345.

85. Marshall VR; Ludbrook J. The relative importance of patient and examiner variability in a test of clinical skills. *Br J Med Educ*; 1972;6:212-217.

86. McClelland DC. Intelligence is not the best predictor of job performance. *J Am Psychol Sci*; 1993;2:5-6.

87. McDermott JF; Tanguay PE; Scheiber SC; Juul D; Shore JH; Tucker GJ; McCurdy L; Terr LC. Reliability of the Part II Board Certification Examination in Psychiatry: Interexaminer Consistency. *Am J Psychiatry*; 1991;148:1672-1674.

88. McGuire CH. The oral examination as a measure of professional competence. *J Med Educ*; 1966;41:267-274.

89. McGuire CH. Studies of the oral examination: Experiences with orthopaedic surgery. In Lloyd JS; Langsley DG (Eds.): *Evaluating the Skills of Medical Specialists.* Evanston, IL: American Board of Medical Specialties; 1983, pp. 105-109.

90. McLean LD; Dauphinee WD; Rotman A. The oral examination in internal medicine of The Royal College of Physicians and Surgeons of Canada: A reliability analysis. Ann R Coll Phys Surg Canada; 1988;21:510-514.

91. Meskauskas JA; Norcini JJ. Standard-setting in written and interactive (oral) specialty certification examinations. *Eval Hlth Prof*; 1980;3:321-360.

92. Meskauskas JA. Studies of the oral examination: The examinations of the subspecialty board of cardiovascular disease of the American Board of Internal Medicine. In Lloyd JS; Langsley DG (Eds.): *Evaluating the Skills of Medical Specialists.* Evanston, IL: American Board of Medical Specialties; 1983, pp. 115-120.

93. Meyerhoff JL; Oleshansky MA; Mougey EH. Psychologic stress increases plasma levels of prolactin, cortisol, and POMC- derived peptides in man. *Psychosom Med*; 1988; 50:295-303.

94. Miller G. The orthopedic training study. *JAMA*; 1968;206:601-606.

95. Moss PA. Shifting conceptions of validity in educational measurement: Implications for performance assessment. *Rev Educ Res*; 1992;62:229-258.

96. Munger B; Maatsch JL. Simulated patient encounters in Emergency Medicine. *Proceedings*, Annenberg Conference on Clinical Skills Assessment. American Medical Association (AMA), National Board of Medical Examiners (NBME), Annenberg Center for Health Sciences at Eisenhower (ACHSE); October 1987, pp. 1-4. (Unpublished Report)

97. Muzzin LJ; Hart L. Oral examinations. In Neufield VR; Norman GR (Eds.): *Assessing Clinical Competence.* New York: Springer Publ Co; 1985, pp. 71-93.

98. Newble DI; Hoare J; Sheldrake PF. The selection and training of examiners for clinical examinations. *Med Educ*; 1980;14:345-349.

99. Nichols PD. A framework for developing cognitively diagnostic assessments. *Rev Educ Res*; 1994;64:575-603.

100. Norcini JJ; Swanson DB; Webster GD. Reliability, validity and efficiency of various item formats in the assessment of physicians. *Proceedings*, Ann Conf Res Med Educ, Assoc Am Med Coll; 1983, 53-58.

101. Norcini JJ; Swanson DB; Grosso LJ; Webster GD. A comparison of several methods for scoring patient management problems. *Proceedings*, Ann Conf Res Med Educ, Assoc Am Med Coll; 1984; 41-46.

102. Norman GR. Defining competence: A methodological review. In Neufeld VR; Norman GR (Eds.): *Assessing clinical competence*. New York: Springer Publ Co; 1985, pp. 15-35.

103. Norman G; Bordage G; Curry L; Dauphinee D; Jolly B; Newble D; Rothman A; Stalenhoef B; Stillman P; Swanson D; Tonesk Z. A review of recent innovations in assessment. In Wakeford R (Ed.): *Directions in Clinical Assessment: Report of the First Cambridge Conference on the Assessment of Clinical Competence*. Cambridge, England: Cambridge Univ Sch Clin Med; Addenbrooke's Hosp, 1985 (pp. 9-27).

104. Norman GR. Striking the balance. *Acad Med*; 1994;69:209-210.

105. Norman GR. Symposium: The essence of clinical competence-psychological studies of expert reasoning in medicine. *Proceedings*, Ann Conf Res Med Educ, Assoc Am Med Coll; 1983;322:278-286.

106. Paese PW; Kinnaly M. Peer input and revised judgment: Exploring the effects of (un)biased confidence. *J Appl Soc Psychol*; 1993;23:1989-2011.

107. Page G; Bordage G. The Medical Council of Canada's Key Features Project: A more valid written examination of clinical decision-making skills. *Acad Med*; 1995;70:104-110.

108. Patel VL; Kaufman DR. On poultry expertise, precocious kids, and diagnostic reasoning. *Acad Med*; 1994;69:971-972.

109. Pietroni M. The assessment of competence in surgical trainees. *Ann R Coll Surg Engl*; 1993;75:200-202.

110. Platt JR. On maximizing the information obtained from science examinations, written and oral. *Am J Physics*; 1961;29:111-122.

111. Pokorny AD; Frazier SH. An evaluation of oral examinations. *J Med Educ*; 1966;41: 28-40.

112. Pope WD. Anaesthesia oral examination. *Can J Anaesth*; 1993;40:907-910.

113. Pressey SL; Pressey LC; Barnes EJ. The final ordeal. *J Higher Educ*; 1932;3:261-264.

114. Price PB; Taylor CW; Richards JM; Jacobsen TL. Measurement of physician performance. *J Med Educ*; 1964;39:203-211.

115. Rakel RE. Defining competence in specialty practice: The need for relevance. In Lloyd JS; Langsley DG (Eds.): *Evaluating the Skills of Medical Specialists*. Evanston, IL: American Board of Medical Specialties; 1983, pp. 85-91.

116. Raymond MR; Webb LC; Houston WM. Correcting performance-rating errors in oral examinations. *Eval Hlth Prof*; 1991;14:100-122.

117. Redelmeier DA; Shafir E. Medical decision making in situations that offer multiple alternatives. *JAMA*; 1995;273:302-305.

118. Ree MJ; Earles JA. G is to psychology, what carbon is to chemistry: A reply to Sternberg and Wagner, McCleland, and Calfee. *Curr Dir Psychol Sci*; 1993;2:11-12.

119. Reed GF. Experience with the patient simulation oral examination procedure, American Board of Otolaryngology. *Proceedings*, Conf Res Eval Proc, Chicago, IL: American Board of Medical Specialties; 1978, pp. 14-20.

120. Regehr G. Chickens and children do not an expert make. *Acad Med*; 1994;69:970-971.

121. Remer R. Improving oral exams - An application of Morenean Sociometry. *J Grp Psychotherapy, Psychodrama and Sociometry*; 1990;43:35-42.

122. Reznick RK; Blackmore D; Cohen R; Baumber J; Rothman A; Smee S; Chalmers A; Poldre P; Birtwhistte R; Walsh P; Spady D; Berard M. An objective structured clinical examination for the licentiate of the Medical Council of Canada: From research to reality. *Acad Med*; 1993;68:S4-S6.

123. Robb KV; Rothman AI. The assessment of clinical skills in general medical residents - Comparison of the objective structured clinical examination to a conventional oral examination. In Lloyd JS; Langsley DG (Eds.): *How to Evaluate Residents*. Evanston, IL: American Board of Medical Specialties; 1986, pp. 325-332.

124. Rosinski EF. The oral examination as an educational assessment procedure. In Lloyd JS; Langsley DG (Eds.): *Evaluating the Skills of Medical Specialists*. Evanston, IL: American Board of Medical Specialties; 1983, pp. 101-104.

125. Rowland-Morin PA; Burchard KW; Garb JL; Coe NP. Influence of effective communication by surgery students on their oral examination scores. *Acad Med*; 1991;66:169-171.

126. Sawa RJ. Assessing interviewing skills: The simulated office oral examination. *J Fam Pract*; 1986;23:567-571.

127. Schmidt FL; Hunter, JE. Tacit knowledge, practical intelligence, general mental ability, and job knowledge. *Curr Dir Psychol Sci*; 1993;2:8-9.

128. Slogoff S; Hughes FP. Validity of scoring 'Dangerous Answers' on a written certification examination. *J Med Educ*; 1987;62:625-631.

129. Solomon DJ; Reinhart MA; Bridgham RG; Munger BS; Starnaman S. An Assessment of an oral examination format for evaluating clinical competence in emergency medicine. *Acad Med*; 1990;65:S43-S44.

130. Stembridge VA. Experiments in revision of the oral examination: American Board of Pathology. In Lloyd JS; Langsley DG (Eds.): *Evaluating the Skills of Medical Specialists.* Evanston, IL: American Board of Medical Specialties; 1983, pp. 133-135.

131. Sternberg RJ; Wagner RK. The g-ocentric view of intelligence and job performance is wrong. *Curr Dir Psychol Sci*; 1993;2:1-5.

132. Stevens WC. Training of oral examiners: The Oral examination workshop of the American Board of Anesthesiology. In JS Lloyd (Ed.): *Oral Examinations in Medical Specialty Board Certification.* Evanston, IL: American Board of Medical Specialties, 73-78.

133. Stillman PL; Regan MB; Haley HL; Norcini JJ; Friedman M; Sutnick AI. The use of a patient note to evaluate clinical skills of first-year residents who are graduates of foreign medical schools. *Acad Med*; 1992;67:S57-S59.

134. Sutnick AI; Stillman PL; Norcini JJ; Friedman M; Regan MB; Williams RG; Kachur EK; Haggerty MA; Wilson MP. ECFMG assessment of clinical competence of graduates of foreign medical schools. *JAMA*; 1993;270:1041-1045.

135. Tamblyn R; Abrahamowicz M; Schnarch B; Colliver JA. Can standardized patients predict real-patient satisfaction with the doctor-patient relationship? *Teach Learn Med*; 1994;6:36-44.

136. Taylor WC; Grace M; Taylor TR; Fincham SM; Skakun EN. The use of computerized patient management problems in a certifying examination. *Med Educ*; 1976;10:179-182.

137. Thomas CS; Mellsop G; Callender K; Crawshaw J; Ellis PM; Hall A; MacDonald J; Silfverskiold P; Romans-Clarkson S. The oral examination: A study of academic and non-academic factors. *Med Educ*; 1992;27:433-439.

138. Trimble OC. The oral examination: Its validity and reliability. *School Society*; 1934;39:550-552.

139. Valberg L; Firstbrook J. A project to improve the measurement of professional competence for specialty certification in Internal Medicine. *Ann R Coll Phys Surg Canada*; 1977; 10:278-282.

140. Van der Vleuten C; Newble D; Case S; Holsgrove G; McCann B; McRae C; Saunders N. Methods of assessment in certification. In Newble D; Jolly B; Wakeford R (Eds.): *The certification and recertification of doctors: Issues in the assessment of clinical competence.* Great Britain: Cambridge Univ Press; 1994, pp. 105-125.

141. Van Rosendaal GMA; Couture AL; Danoff DS; Hollomby DJ; Turnbull JM. The Royal College examination in internal medicine: Where to from here? *Ann R Coll Phys Surg Canada*; 1994;27:216-218.

142. Van Wart AD. A problem-solving oral examination for Family Medicine. *J Med Educ*; 1974;49:673-680.

143. Vassend O. Examination stress, personality and self-reported physical symptoms. *Scand J Psychol*; 1988;29:21-32.

144. Wainer H; Wang XB; Thissen D. How well can we compare scores on test forms that are constructed by examinees' choice? *J Educ Meas*; 1994;31: 183-199.

145. Waugh D; Moyse CA. Medical Education II: Oral examinations: A video study of the reproducibility of grades in pathology. *Can Med Assoc J*; 1969;100:635-640.

146. Wigton RC. The effects of student personal characteristics on the evaluation of clinical performance. *J Med Educ*; 1980;55:423-427.

147. Wilson GM; Harden R; Lever R; Robertson J; MacRitchie J. Examination of clinical examiners. *Lancet*; 1969;1:37-40.

148. Woolliscroft JO; Swanson DB; Case SM. Validity of extended matching and short answer response formats with pattern recognition items. In Harden RM; Hart IR; Mulholland H (Eds.) *International Conference Proceedings*: Approaches to the assessment of clinical competence. Dundee, Scottish Centre for Medical Education: 1992, pp. 459-464.

149. Yang JC; Laube DW. Improvement of reliability of an oral examination by a structured evaluation instrument. *J Med Educ*; 1983;58:864-872.

150. Zaglaniczny KL. Council on certification professional practice analysis. *J Am Assoc Nurse Anesthetists*; 1993;61:241-255.

Author Index

Subject Index